An Introduction to
WRITING *for*
HEALTH
PROFESSIONALS

the
SMART
way

FOURTH EDITION

An Introduction to

WRITING *for*
HEALTH
PROFESSIONALS

the
SMART
way

Glennis Zilm
BSN, BJ, MA, LittD (H)

Beth Perry
RN, PhD

ELSEVIER

VP Education Content: Kevonne Holloway
Content Strategist (Acquisitions): Roberta A. Spinosa-Millman
Content Development Specialist: Theresa Fitzgerald
Publishing Services Manager: Unni Deepthi
Project Manager: Radjan Lourde Selvanadin
Copy Editor: Christina Schwaller
Book Designer: Renee Duenow
Typesetting and Assembly: SPi Global

Working together
to grow libraries in
developing countries

www.elsevier.com • www.bookaid.org

1 2 3 4 5 6 7 8 9

3 citations, references, and bibliographies, 47

4 common errors in writing, 82

The purpose of good writing is to communicate ideas effectively—and effectively usually means as clearly and concisely as possible. Some writers forget this simple goal when they sit down to write. Others neglect this goal because they wish to impress readers with what they believe will be dramatic effects. The need for effective written communications in today's business world, including the health care system, has never been greater. Because of this, all health professionals must be able to write well.

This book is intended to be a beginner's guide for students entering the health professions who are having or believe they will have difficulties with written assignments. You probably have the ability to prepare academic papers, but you may have forgotten some of the basic rules you learned in high school. You may be at a different stage in the development of your writing skills and have problems different from those of your classmates. For example, you may love to write and like to take a highly creative approach but find your instructors do not appreciate this. You may have taken several English courses already or may be taking writing courses concurrently but find that some of the rules from these courses do not apply to the style of writing used by health professionals.

This small "how to" book encourages you to write "The SMART Way." Exercises scattered throughout the chapters allow you to recognize problem areas in your own writing. Each chapter concludes with a brief list of points to remember and a list of the references used in the preparation of that chapter. These are set using APA style to give you more examples of a bibliography. In Chapter 1, you examine the essential elements of communication—Source * Message * Audience * Route * Tone—and learn how to apply them.

In Chapter 2, you learn to use the acronym PROCESS, which shows a series of steps to help you organize content more easily and write more quickly and effectively. Although the messages in these opening chapters may seem relatively simple, application of these skills can change your approach to writing and enable you to improve as a writer throughout your career.

In Chapter 3, the focus is on finding and properly citing information and on references and bibliographies. A few comments are offered on plagiarism, which is a growing problem on campuses. You likely learned about these topics in high school, but they are much more important in the kind of writing you are expected to do for college and university communications. Lessons on the use of references and bibliographies are taught in many first-year, elective arts courses. If you have not taken such courses, this will be an essential chapter. Your instructors usually expect you to have sound bibliographical skills and to develop them further with every paper you write. You should begin by reading the first three chapters carefully, completing the exercises as you go along.

In Chapter 4, you review some common errors that health professionals—and many other writers—make, and you learn how to avoid them. This book is not intended to replace a full-credit course in grammar and writing skills; it is intended to help high school graduates avoid errors that abound in academic and business writing. All of these common errors apply to student papers, which is what this book is about. We then provide, in Appendix A, an example of a student paper that illustrates this information.

Chapter 5 illustrates how you can use the first four chapters as a base for other written communications, such as documentation and charting, business letters, memos, electronic communications, class presentations, résumés and curriculum vitae, minutes and agendas, research papers, theses and dissertations, and articles.

The final chapter, Chapter 6, briefly recaps many of the important themes developed in the book.

Appendix A may be one of the most useful sections of this book for many beginning students. It contains a guide to the format, layout, and structure of a first-year student paper as recommended by the manuals of the American Psychological Association (APA); this is the style guide most commonly used in health disciplines and in journals for health professionals. Most health professional programs require students to learn and use APA style for references and bibliographies. Appendix A features a nursing example, but it also gives background details and illustrates the most common types of references you will use in papers, especially during early courses. This brief guide does not replace APA manuals, but it should be sufficient to help you thoroughly understand basic reference and citation styles and learn how to use APA manuals more efficiently.

We hope you will find the design of this new edition lively, functional, and easy to use. For example, at various points in the book, the designers have set portions in a distinctive colour. These features are intended to draw your attention to student examples that follow the formatting, spelling, capitalization, punctuation, and other points of style recommended by APA. As explained in this book, APA style is the one usually recommended for student papers in programs for health professionals. Please note that the text portions of this book follow the "house style" established by Elsevier (the publisher) and that Elsevier's house style sometimes differs from APA style.

A comprehensive Evolve Web site (http://evolve.elsevier.com/Zilm/SMART/) is also featured in conjunction with this edition; it provides further resources and can be reached through the Elsevier website. Students who want more exercises than are provided in the text will find additional Review Questions on the student portion of the site. Also included are more examples of APA citations, a Guide to APA Style in Reference Lists and Bibliographies, Tips for Writing Well, and Writing Resources. In both the student resources area and the instructor resource area, a section appears featuring answers to Frequently Asked Questions as well as ways to communicate your suggestions and comments to us. The instructor portion of the site offers PPT slides, Marking Symbols, Reading Resources, and Tips for Marking.

Literally hundreds of students and health professionals have used *The SMART Way* throughout the years and report that it has helped them to become better writers and communicators. We hope you, too, will find it useful in all your writing.

reviewers

Lori Carre, RN, BScN, MN
Professor, School of Health Sciences
Seneca College of Applied Arts &
  Technology
Barrie, Ontario

Jane Clifford O'Brien,
  PhD, MS, EdL, OTR/L, FAOTA
Professor, Occupational Therapy
Department of Occupational
  Therapy
University of New England
Portland, Maine

Michelle A. Connell,
  RN, BScN, MEd
Nursing Professor,
Ryerson, Centennial and George
  Brown Collaborative Nursing
  Degree Program
School of Community and Health
  Studies
Centennial College
Toronto, Ontario

Shannon Kenrick-Rochon,
  BScN, MN, NP-PHC
Professor
Cambrian College
Sudbury, Ontario

Tania Kristoff, RN, MN
Assistant Professor
College of Nursing
University of Saskatchewan
Prince Albert, Saskatchewan

Nadine Nadalutti,
  RN, BNSc, MEAE
Coordinator, Practical Nurse
  Program
Columbia College
Calgary, Alberta

Angela M. Spencer, BS, MHA
Chicago Community Learning
  Centre
Chicago, Illinois

GLENNIS ZILM, now semiretired, has combined her nursing background with journalism for more than 50 years. Since 2003, she has been an honorary professor in the University of British Columbia School of Nursing. A graduate in nursing from UBC, she also has degrees in journalism and communications. A former assistant editor of *Canadian Nurse* and managing editor of *B.C. Medical Journal*, she worked for five years with the Canadian Press in Edmonton and Ottawa, as well as in radio and television in Vancouver before becoming a full-time freelance writer, editor, and consultant, mainly in health disciplines. She gave writing workshops to nurses and other health professionals, and, as a guest lecturer, taught nursing and writing skills courses at universities and colleges across Canada. In 2006, she received an honorary Doctor of Letters from Kwantlen University College. One of Glennis Zilm's major interests is the history of nursing. She is co-author, with Ethel Warbinek, of *Legacy: History of Nursing Education at the University of British Columbia, 1919–1994*, and co-author, with Sheila Zerr and Valerie Grant, of a scholarly biography, *Labor of Love: A Memoir of Gertrude Richards Ladner 1879 to 1976*. In 2004, she was awarded the John B. Neilson Award by Associated Medical Services, Inc., of Toronto, for her "high level of contributions to the teaching, research, publication, and preservation of nursing history."

The "SMART Way" principles are based on insights gained during her graduate studies in communications. These insights were sharpened during workshops and while teaching courses at various colleges and universities across Canada, and especially during the introduction of distance education programs for nurses.

BETH PERRY is a professor in the Faculty of Health Disciplines at Athabasca University. Beth is a registered nurse and completed her doctorate in educational administration at the University of Alberta. Her dissertation on exemplary nursing care was published by the Canadian Nurses Association in a book titled *Moments in Time: Images of Exemplary Nursing*. Beth discovered her passion for words and writing while using phenomenology as the methodology for her doctoral work and since has written multiple books and papers featuring stories and poetry that convey the essence of humanity within the limitation of words. As a professor she has guided graduate students through the arduous process of thesis work and embraces the opportunity to teach writing skills alongside research prowess. Teaching online has sharpened her interest in effective electronic communications, and Beth is currently completing a second project funded by the Social Sciences and Humanities Research Council of Canada; the project focuses on engaging online learners through arts-based teaching strategies, including stories, poetry, and dramatic approaches. She is co-author of *Teaching Health Professionals Online: Frameworks and Strategies*. In 2015, Beth received the Canadian Association of Schools of Nursing award for excellence in nursing education. Along with a colleague, she received the Commonwealth of Learning award for excellence in distance education in 2013. In 2017, she co-authored a chapter in an award-winning book, *Emergence and Innovation in Digital Learning*.

Throughout the years, many talented individuals have assisted in the development of workshops, distance education manuals, and this book, and we thank them. As well, many thanks to the hundreds of students who were part of the evolution of this book.

We would like to thank Roberta A. Spinosa-Millman and Laurie Gower of Elsevier for their enthusiasm and editorial support, as well as our developmental editor Theresa Fitzgerald for her expert guidance and her assistance in navigating us through the challenging waters of publication today.

Glennis owes special thanks to Valerie and Keith Chapman and the rest of her family for patience, support, understanding, and encouragement, especially during the rewriting and polishing steps—which, as in all writing, take more time than one anticipates.

Beth thanks her husband Otto Mahler for technical support in navigating the perpetually changing online world and her doctoral supervisor Dr. Eugene Ratsoy for modelling the power of precise word choice and perfect punctuation.

Written communications form a major part of the glue that helps people work together cooperatively, harmoniously, and effectively. Written communications are vital in hospitals and other health agencies, and all health professionals must be able to write well. In modern agencies, writing, including that via electronic media, is often the only practical method of communication. Most health professionals, even those doing mainly clinical care, spend 10 to 40% of their work time writing. Managers spend even more time than that. Furthermore, as interrelationships grow among health professionals, agencies, and community- and home-based care workers, written communications will likely increase.

Because your instructors know this, they want you to develop your writing skills, and usually a portion of an assignment mark is based on your ability to write well. Your writing must be clear (i.e., organized and well expressed, with good grammar and punctuation) so the content of the paper will be clear. Most programs for health professionals do not include courses on how to write. You are expected to bring with you the sound, basic skills you learned in high school; you may even be required to pass a college-entry examination to show that your writing skills are at that level. You are also expected to improve these skills as you progress through your program. By the end of your courses, you are expected to have reached the scholarly level of college and university graduates. Usually, you must do this mainly through your own efforts. For this reason, many students opt to take elective courses in academic writing or in business English.

Some courses will focus on ways to improve your oral communication skills, especially in one-on-one communications (e.g., nurse-to-patient or therapist-to-nurse). And some of your courses will devote time to the specifics of documentation in your discipline (e.g., charting). Fortunately, there are principles that work in all communication. The first step to good writing is to understand the five basic elements that affect all methods of communication (oral, written, musical, visual, physical [i.e. body language], electronic, and so on). These five elements can be organized using the SMART acronym:

Source * **M**essage * **A**udience * **R**oute * **T**one

Understanding these elements of communication and their interrelationships will help you to:

- recognize your strengths and work on your weaknesses;
- identify your objectives and clearly state your message;
- identify, understand, and respond to readers' needs;
- select the most appropriate method of communication (oral presentation, essay, memo, email, letter, report, brief, review article, proposal, or other); and
- select the appropriate tone for the communication.

This breakdown of any single communication into these five basic elements may sound simple, but it really is not. $E = mc^2$ sounds simple, too, but that formula represents Einstein's theory of relativity! The important thing is that you understand and use the basic elements of communication.

The five elements integrate to form one package, and you cannot isolate any one element (see Figure 1.1). Similarly, when you are baking, once you blend flour, sweetener, liquid, and fat, you cannot remove any one of them from the mixture. Those four basic ingredients illustrate another factor related to communication principles: they are basic elements of crepes, pancakes, scones, and pound cake, but whether you get crepes or cakes depends on the relative amounts of those ingredients. Furthermore, you can vary the ingredients: you can use whole wheat flour, honey, skim milk, and oil, or you can use cake flour, white sugar, cream, and butter. The outcome will reflect the knowledge you have about the ingredients, how to mix them, how to cook them, and how to present them. The same applies in writing. So let us examine those five essential SMART elements before we start to mix them.

SOURCE

When you read a front-page newspaper headline that says "Student Fees to Increase," you immediately wonder "Who says so?" If the source for that comment is a visiting pop star, you may smile and treat the story somewhat lightly. If, however, the source is the president of your college or university,

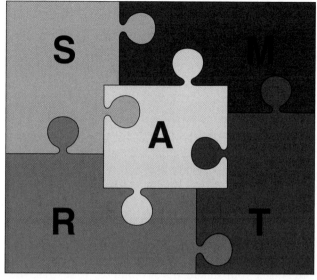

FIGURE 1.1 The SMART Elements

you begin to worry about having to pay more fees. You, the reader, are influenced by the source.

If you are looking through a professional journal, such as *Canadian Nurse* or *American Pharmacy*, and you see a title that applies to your topic, you should assess who wrote the article by looking at the author note that is usually on the first page or at the end. If the author is someone who works in the discipline, or if the remarks indicate the authors did research on the topic, this article may have more credible information than one written by a student or a nonprofessional. Articles written by students or by patients may still be valid, but you must weigh the qualifications and experiences of the source because these affect the content.

Similarly, when you are the writer (source), your readers need to know your qualifications. Before you begin to write, ask yourself, "What are my qualifications for this communication?" You need to weigh your qualifications for preparing the communication. Before you begin to write, ask yourself, "What are my qualifications for this communication?"

You may have experiences that give you knowledge about the subject. For example, if you are asked to write a paper on care of older adults and you have lived with grandparents for several years, you have personal knowledge about challenges people may face as they grow older. If the topic for a paper is early human development and you have cared for children, you have likely observed something about developmental stages. If you are asked to write on environmental concerns and you had a summer job in a recycling depot, you may have practical knowledge about landfill sites and composting habits. If you have diabetes, you bring a different perspective to a paper on this topic than if you have never known anyone with the condition. So you can draw on your own experiences.

Furthermore, once you have had several classes on a subject and have read the textbooks, the instructor will expect you to have absorbed the basic concepts behind the course. For example, if you have completed several nursing courses, you are expected to have more knowledge about anatomy, physiology, and health needs than the average non-nurse. When you write papers for instructors, they expect a level of basic expertise based on all your courses. But does taking one course or reading a book make you an expert in the subject area? If you are not an expert (as will be the case when you are writing most student papers), then you may have to draw on the findings of researchers to bolster your statements or opinions. To do this, you need to know how to use electronic and print resources to find information and how to use references in your papers so that your remarks are credible. Much more information on appropriate use and citation of resources is available in Chapter 3.

Sometimes you will have views of your own, even strong opinions, that should be included in your paper. In some assignments, your instructor will ask you to give your own views. However, you must still be able to substantiate them (give illustrations drawn from your experience) and expound on the reasons or rationales for your views. As well, you may need to show how your views compare with the "accepted wisdom" or traditional views on the subject, which may mean reading widely to identify where your views agree with or differ from those of others. When you bring in supporting comments, you also have to judge whether the experts that you are using are credible and well researched.

You also need to know other things about yourself as a source. As well as your knowledge of the subject, you need to know your strengths and weaknesses as a writer. Think about yourself as a writer. Do you have good writing skills? Can you identify your strengths and weaknesses? The statements in Exercise 1.1, which are based on comments by students in writing skills workshops, may help you to identify your strengths and weaknesses.

Exercise 1.1 Self-Assessment

All writers have problem areas—even professional writers. However, professional writers have learned to recognize their problems and to concentrate on overcoming them. You need to know yourself. Once you have identified your problems, you can begin to solve them. First, take a minute and write down what you think are **your** *three* most important **strengths and weaknesses** related to your writing.

Strengths	Weaknesses
_____	_____
_____	_____
_____	_____

Now that you have identified what you believe are **your** strengths and weaknesses, look at the following list of 15 comments. These were typical comments made by students in writing skills classes when they were asked to list their strengths and weaknesses. Think about each comment carefully and then tick it if you believe it applies to you. Then also tick the box in the next column if you think it might be a comment routinely made by other students in your courses.

	Typical of Me	Typical of Others
1. I have difficulty expressing my thoughts.	❏	❏
2. I dislike writing and put it off until the last minute.	❏	❏
3. I like to share my views with others.	❏	❏
4. I have problems finding information on the topic.	❏	❏
5. I like to read widely on a subject.	❏	❏
6. I like to write.	❏	❏
7. I have difficulty finding time to write.	❏	❏
8. I like to write first thing in the morning (or late at night, or other special time).	❏	❏
9. I have difficulty getting started when I finally do sit down to write.	❏	❏
10. I do not know the correct form that my written communication should take.	❏	❏
11. I usually start working on an assignment the night before it is due.	❏	❏
12. When I get started, I tend to be too wordy, too verbose, and my paper is too long.	❏	❏

	Typical of Me	Typical of Others
13. When I get started, I tend to be too blunt, too brusque, and my paper usually is too short.	❑	❑
14. My writing is rambling and usually lacks a sense of focus.	❑	❑
15. I have difficulty with basic grammar, spelling, or punctuation.	❑	❑

COMMENTS ON SELF-ASSESSMENT EXERCISE 1.1

The comments are based on those of health professionals, including students, who participated in various writing workshops over two decades. Workshop participants indicated responses in classes by a show of hands, and reported data are based on informal records kept over the years. Go over the comments carefully, concentrating on areas that are challenging to you.

Just having thought out your responses in Exercise 1.1 may have been enlightening for you. When you examine these common comments, you will notice that many are matters of organization and time management rather than problems with writing, although these definitely affect a person's ability to write well! Here are the workshop comments about these strengths and weaknesses:

1. In the workshops, about 65% of participants indicated that they have difficulty expressing themselves. Surprisingly, most participants (up to 90% in some workshops) said they believe that others do not have this problem. You can take some solace in the thought that you are not alone—writing is hard work for most people.

2. Almost everyone dislikes writing and tends to put it off. Professional writers overcome this block by setting deadlines and learning to stick to them. Ways to deal with procrastination are addressed in the following chapters, especially Chapter 2.

3. Many people like to share their views, so this can be a real strength. Sharing your views will help you to get started with a writing project.

4. Finding information about a topic on which you must write is always a problem. Chapters 2 and 3 contain more on this. Start thinking about your ability to locate and use credible print and electronic resources. Although you may have learned how to use these resources in high school, you may find that health professionals take a different approach. You will need to learn digital literacy skills to guide you to locate,

evaluate, and use information effectively. There is more on this subject in Chapter 3.

5. Reading widely on a subject is an important strength for those taking academic courses because instructors may provide massive reading lists. Reading the articles and textbooks required for the course is a splendid way to gather information.

6. If you like to write, you are indeed a rare individual. (Even well-known novelists admit that they like being a writer but hate to write.) But do you only like to write about topics of your own choosing? Most of the writing that you are required to do as a student or in the professional world does not fall into this category. Often you must write what readers want or need to know rather than allow yourself to do creative writing. This point is covered more fully in this chapter in the section titled Audience.

7. About 40% of workshop participants said that finding time to write is a major problem. Much learning at the postsecondary level is self-directed; for every hour of course time a student should spend three additional hours reading, writing, and thinking about (or discussing) course material. If finding time to write is your major problem, you may need a time management course rather than a writing course. Just being aware that you have a problem is a great starting point for improvement. Good writing takes time—even for professionals. You may need to book "writing time" into your organizer, because scheduling helps. Consider doing so if you tend to leave an assignment until the night before it is due. Even if you are a superb writer, you cannot do a good job if you are rushed. There is more on this topic in Chapter 2.

8. One small, but important, point to consider is the time of day that you like to write. Some people like to write first thing in the morning; if this is your style, then find a quiet room at home where you can write from 6 to 8 A.M. Others like to write in the evening, which may be a problem if it conflicts with family time. If so, you may need to move your workspace to another area of the house or plan to spend a couple of evenings a week working elsewhere.

9. Almost everyone has difficulty getting started, although two-thirds of workshop participants do not see others as having this common problem. Chapter 2 contains more on this point. The best way to start is to go to your computer and apply the seat of your pants to the seat of your chair.

10. Two major reasons for this book are to help students learn the correct format for written communications, whether papers, reports, articles, or

email, and to help students use references accurately. These topics are addressed in Chapters 3 and 5.

11. If leaving an assignment until the last minute is your problem, please change your approach. College and university papers require a great deal of reading and research, and you need to start planning your paper the day you receive the assignment. See Chapter 2 for more information on how to deal with this habit.

12 & 13. In the workshops, about 60 to 70% of participants said they believe that their writing is "long-winded." However, only about 30% believe that others have this problem. A much smaller number—about 10%—of participants believe that their writing is too blunt or too direct or that they cannot make a letter, report, or assignment long enough. In Chapter 2, you will find more on the importance of envisioning the length (or word count) of the finished document even as you begin writing the first sentence.

14. About 35% of participants said a major problem is that their writing is "too rambling" or that they cannot focus the message. Chapter 2 offers suggestions to resolve this problem. About 50% often find that the writing of others rambles—even in the articles assigned as required readings. Rambling makes content unclear, so you do need to concentrate on improving this area of your writing.

15. The final item in Exercise 1.1 concerns actual writing problems (rather than with time management, for instance). You may need to improve your skills in grammar, punctuation, and spelling. Usually, only 10 to 15% of students believe that they have difficulty with basic grammar and punctuation. However, instructors report that student assignments contain serious errors in these areas. You may believe that grammar and punctuation are not important, but college and university graduates are expected to achieve high standards in these areas. People do care about grammar, punctuation, and spelling; for example, a book on punctuation—*Eats, Shoots & Leaves* by Lynne Truss (2004)—became a worldwide bestseller.

Grammar, punctuation, and spelling mistakes are more common when students rush through the final draft of a paper. About 80% of students admit that they have difficulty with spelling. Computer spell-checkers help, but you need access to a good dictionary as well. You should also know that business leaders and college or university instructors get upset about spelling errors in material that they have to read. Instructors, even if they, too, have difficulty with spelling, often take off marks for spelling errors in student papers; the rationale is that spelling errors or typing errors (called "typos") indicate a sloppy, rushed presentation. Problems with basic grammar, punctuation, and spelling are much more common than you may believe—and can seriously affect your marks! These problems are addressed in Chapter 4.

<u>M</u>ESSAGE

The second element in the SMART acronym is the message: the content of your communication; the information being conveyed. Although the message is the most important part of almost every communication, it will be affected by the other basic elements. Because of this, you need to know exactly what your message is—you need to work out what you want to say *before* you begin to write. This means you have to do a lot of thinking and planning beforehand. This thinking process is the hardest part of writing.

Knowing what you want to say helps you choose how to convey your message. For example, if you merely want to say "hello" and remind your mother that you are thinking of her, then you may not need to write a formal letter; a text message might do, or a telephone call might be better. Some messages are best delivered face to face. If you want to give a patient instructions about rehabilitation after an operation, then sitting down and having a conversation might do. You may also want to write out the instructions in point form, or find an instruction sheet issued by your agency to complement and reinforce verbal instructions. Written instructions, whether hardcopy or electronic, have many advantages because they can be kept and referred to later.

During your academic courses, you will often be asked to prepare written assignments. Sometimes the assignment topic will be given to you by the instructor. For example, if you are asked to read and comment on an article or articles, the instructor may ask you to "compare and contrast the points raised," or to "summarize the article in your own words," or to "choose your own topic." These requirements mean entirely different things, and if you do not follow the instructions in your message, you will lose marks.

Before you can begin to write, however, you must identify what you want or need to say. You want your message in every written communication to be clear, concise, logically presented, accurate, well researched, and appropriate. Chapter 2 contains more information on planning and organizing the message.

Your message affects all other elements in the SMART acronym, too. For example, for some messages, it may be more appropriate to use a song or poem than a formal paper. If you want your message to reach a certain demographic or population, the reading level and medium of the message needs to be carefully chosen. Sometimes, "digital natives" (those who are technically literate from an early age) may be most successfully reached with a message presented in 250 characters or less.

AUDIENCE

Just as it is important that you know and understand the source and the message, you also need to know exactly to whom a communication is directed: the audience. If you are talking to a child who is your patient, you use different words and explain your message differently than if you are talking to a colleague. So when you sit down to write, you need to visualize exactly who will receive your communication. Other textbook authors refer to this person as the "receiver" or the "reader," but all experts agree that you need to think about the audience for your communications.

Most student assignments are prepared for an audience of one person (the course instructor), so you have to consider the specific knowledge, skills, and expectations of that individual. This does not mean that you must kowtow to or play up to the teacher, just that you need to be aware of what your instructor has covered in class and what you are expected to know or to learn. If your instructor supports one position and you are going to propose another view, you will need to anticipate questions your instructor might raise. Do not assume your instructor knows what you mean; if you do, you may omit important pieces of the explanation. Remember, too, that instructors in psychology or law or anthropology may not be familiar with terms you use regularly in health disciplines; you may need to use a slightly different vocabulary in these courses.

Sometimes your instructor will ask you to write an assignment for a specific audience, such as a letter to the editor or an instruction guide for patients. Sometimes you are preparing information for your classmates or colleagues. If you are emailing a friend, then again you have a different audience and would use a different tone than you would in a report to an agency.

Frequently, instructors clearly spell out points they want you to cover in your assignments. They may tell you the expected word count for the paper. Usually they specify which style manual to use; the *Publication Manual of the American Psychological Association* (APA, 2010) is used throughout the health disciplines, but occasionally style requirements change depending on the audience or route. You need to consider these points. If your instructor has not stipulated an audience, you may need to indicate, early in the assignment, the audience *you* visualized. For example, in a review of a research paper, you might include: "This article is excellent for patients but does not contain enough detail for health professionals."

Audience may also mean a need to adjust to the locale. Vocabulary and spellings may change according to country. For example, if you were in Britain, you might say: "I walked in off the street to the main floor and took the lift up one level to the flat on the first floor." In North America, you would be more likely to say: "I walked in off the street to the first floor and took the elevator up one flight to the apartment on the second floor." Both sentences would mean the same thing. Similarly, spellings may differ by country. As you may notice as you read this book, we use such spellings as *practise* (verb), *analyse* (verb), *humour*, and *colour* and use double consonants in the middle of such words as *levelling* and *modelling*, but not in *focusing* or *biased*. This is because we are Canadian authors writing for an international publisher and our head office is in Toronto. In the United States, the more common spellings would be *practice* (verb and noun), *analyze*, *humor*, and *color*; double consonants are rarely used in the middle of words such as *leveling*, *modeling*, and *focusing*. So you need to be aware of your audience, but, as we will explain more in Chapters 2 and 4, you need to be aware of language distinctions and be consistent within your message.

ROUTE

The route you select to get your message across to the audience is also a vital element, and it, too, is affected by the other SMART elements. The route can vary considerably. For example, you can choose a song, letter, blog, report, play, television show, brief, pamphlet, website, or novel to convey your message. Your instructor will not appreciate these routes, however, if he or she has requested a written essay of 2000 words. There are even different kinds of routes within written assignments (e.g., essay, review, report, article, or personal journal).

Each route has its own format and therefore its own rules. For example, suppose you want to send a short written communication to a friend. Would you use flowered stationery, a business letterhead, a note card, a postcard, or an email? The rules vary for each different route. If it is a friendly, gossipy letter, you might like to use perfumed paper and print with purple ink, but these choices would not be appropriate if your friend works as a personnel officer and you are asking for a job interview.

Keep in mind that writing for social media and academic writing are different. First, your audience is likely to be different. You write scholarly academic papers for an audience of one: your instructor. When you write for social media, you are writing for a broad audience, which often includes the general public. And you may even hope that your message goes viral to reach a huge audience. Second, the topic (message) you write about may be different. When you write academic papers, your instructors may ask you to use resources, such as published research, to support your ideas, or to critique certain ideas using existing knowledge. For social media, the message may not be so precise; it can be any topic that will attract the greatest readership and it is often based on personal experience rather than research. Third, the language tones are different; language used in academic writing is more formal and may include technical words and, sometimes, discipline-specific jargon (see the next section on tone). When you are writing for social media, your purpose is to connect with people from various backgrounds and the language you use is likely more informal. Your goal may be to generate a large following of readers, thus your topic, language, and writing style is likely friendly, approachable, or even provocative. As well, you need to be careful about using social media to send a message that is intended for just your own close circle of friends; once the message is posted to the public it may have unexpected consequences— and follow you throughout your career.

A special route for health professionals concerns patient documentation within agencies, such as electronic medical records (EMRs) or charting; at least one of your courses will cover this route in detail. The SMART principles also apply to these communications, but some rules are entirely different. More details about principles of documentation and charting are located in Chapter 5. You also will likely learn in one of your courses about the nonverbal messages you send when you are talking with someone. Nonverbal messages are conveyed by how you stand, by whether you smile as you talk, and even by what you wear (a business suit versus a clown suit). You also send nonverbal clues about yourself and your written message through choices such as paper or font type, or whether you use emojis in your assignments. If your message is handwritten with a dull pencil on a yellow sticky note and attached to your assignment, then it conveys nonverbal messages to the audience (your instructor), such as "This message was rushed and is not important." A poorly written, last-minute email requesting an assignment extension conveys lack of planning (unless you are sending it from the emergency department where they are tending to your broken leg).

The rules for the presentation of assignment papers at the college and university level are complicated. These may seem like minor considerations, but they are designed to make life easier for instructors (or editors when you are ready to write for professional journals), who often must review dozens, even hundreds, of papers. The rules are so complex that entire books are written about them.

These books are called style manuals, and they are among the important writing tools you need to access. Although many good style manuals are available, the *Publication Manual of the American Psychological Association* (APA, 2010) is most commonly used in most health discipline programs. Other courses, such as English, history, or biology, may call for other style manuals to be used, such as the *MLA Handbook* (Modern Language Association, 2016) or *A Manual for Writers of Research Papers, Theses, and Dissertations: Chicago Style for Students and Researchers* (Turabian, 2018). You should always be certain that you are using the most current editions, some of which are available only in online versions. Some colleges and universities produce their own style guides, which are recommended for their students. You need to find out which manual is recommended for students in your discipline and for courses you may take through other departments. Some instructors give detailed directions on the style they expect you to follow. These instructions may be given on the assignment sheets or in the course syllabus. These specific requirements from the instructor (your audience) override all others.

All style manuals focus on details concerning presentation of a written communication, such as how wide to make margins or what font to use. Other details concern where to place subheadings, when to use capital letters (e.g., sometimes only for the first letter in a book title), how to punctuate when there are options, how to set up a table, when to use numerals and abbreviations (e.g., "10" versus "ten"; "hrs" versus "hours"), how to present quotations, and, most important, how to cite your references.

The *Publication Manual of the American Psychological Association*—or *APA Manual*, as it is commonly called—is widely used for professional health publications. Much information related to APA style is also available on the Internet. If you are a first- or second-year student, you may not need a print copy of the *APA Manual* and can rely on credible online resources. You may wish to purchase a full version, which will help you throughout your career. If you are planning to buy, be sure to get the latest edition; do not get a second-hand copy of an earlier edition. By the time you graduate, you will be as familiar with this book as with a dictionary. In Chapter 3, we review the main points of style you need for your early courses and describe how to use a manual as a reference tool.

You are often required (as in the *APA Manual*) to format your paper using a standard size font with a "serif" (or little line at the bottom of the letter), such as Times New Roman (Courier or Pica) as opposed to a "sans-serif font," such as Arial or Helvetica. Box 1.1 provides examples.

Other style considerations include width of margins, line spacing, size and placement of headings, numbering of pages, and placement of page numbers. Style for headings and subheadings can be complicated; information on APA style for headings is provided in Box 1.2 and you can refer to the sample student paper in Appendix A for more information on headings for assignments.

BOX 1.1   Serif and Sans Serif Fonts

```
Courier is a typeface with serifs.
```
Arial is a sans serif typeface.

BOX 1.2   Headings Using APA Style

Level One Headings

This is the primary heading that would be used, for example, for the title of your paper. Notice that it is centred and uses bold type, it has initial letters of main words capitalized, and it does not end with a period. A centred heading is usually used only once.

APA also recommends using these levels of headings to submit manuscripts for articles going to professional journals, although editors determine the final style used. Just think about articles that you have seen in journals, and you will recall that many of these titles are set in a larger font.

Level Two Headings

Level two headings are flush left and boldface with initial letters of main words capitalized. Note also that there is no extra line of space (i.e., a quadruple space) between the sections in the article.

Level three headings. The third level is indented (using the tab key), bold, and capitalizes only the first word and any proper nouns. It ends with a period and the text starts immediately following the heading. This level is also sometimes known as a paragraph heading (but there may be more than one paragraph following).

Level four headings. It also is indented, boldface, but it appears in italics; the text continues.

Level five headings. Similar to level four headings, but without the boldface font.

TONE

In addition to considering source, message, audience, and route, you need to consider the tone you will use as you write your message. Tone is influenced by all the other elements. It varies along a continuum from informal to formal, and covers the emotional depth you wish to create as you write. For example, do you need to be dictatorial or coaxing? Do you wish to seem harsh and strident or pleasant and gracious? These represent variations in tone. You can be argumentative, persuasive, happy, sad, humorous, positive, negative, or sensitive, depending on the words you choose and the way you arrange them.

The poet Robert Frost knew the importance of tone. He recognized that the inflection of a voice often means more than words. If you word your sentences carefully, you can indicate inflections. An important factor in determining tone is learning to "listen with your mind's ear" as you write. If you listen to your sentences as you write, you will usually achieve the tone you wish to create, as in the following simple examples:

> "Nurse," he whispered, "I think I'm bleeding."
> He shouted, "Nurse, I think I'm bleeding."
> "I think I'm bleeding, Nurse," he snarled.

The position of words within a sentence often helps to create emphasis and set the tone, as in the following:

> Inactivity, poor nutrition, and incontinence predispose patients to skin breakdown.
> Patients are predisposed to skin breakdown through inactivity, poor nutrition, and incontinence.

In the first example, listing the causes at the beginning of the sentence gives them greater impact in a written presentation. Depending on the purpose of the sentence within the rest of the paragraph, this positioning might be preferred. However, listing the causes at the end of the sentence gives them more emphasis and makes them more memorable, so this version may be preferred for an oral presentation.

Deciding what tone to use helps you to select words and phrases as you write. Consider the following:

> "Hey, dude, meet my old man!"
> "Joe, I'd like you to meet my husband."
> "Professor Smith, I would like to introduce my husband."
> "Your Excellency, please allow me to present my spouse."

Tone creates personality in your paper. You can be bland and boring, or you can be exciting and refreshing. Tone is affected by source, message, audience, and route, and you achieve it through your choice of words (vocabulary), as shown above. This choice includes proper use of professional terms (e.g., "pain in the lower right quadrant of the abdomen" versus "tummy ache"). Being respectful is one of the most important points to keep in mind. Instructors frequently tell us that a polite tone is important; blunt emails can show lack of respect. For example, "Send me the password" comes across as brusque and almost rude, while "Dear Professor, if it doesn't inconvenience you too much, when you have time, if you could please send me the password to allow me to access the student exercises I would be forever grateful" is excessive. Out of courtesy, you should also include an informative subject line and set up a digital signature so that your full name and contact information are easily accessible to those you are messaging.

Depending on the degree of formality required, you need to decide whether to use contractions (e.g., *isn't* versus *is not*). Most college papers are expected to be fairly formal in tone, so you would avoid using contractions, which are generally considered informal. Of course, if you are writing dialogue or quoting speech, you would include contractions to indicate that this portion of your paper is intended to be informal.

The use of first-person pronouns (*I/we, my/our, mine/ours*) also affects tone. In extremely formal presentations, writers refer to themselves in the third person (e.g., "Miss Smith regrets she cannot attend His Excellency's reception" versus "I am sorry that I cannot attend the reception," or "This author believes …" rather than "I believe …"). The use of first-person pronouns is permissible in formal writing today, although a few instructors (consider your audience) still prefer that you do not use them. For example, you should use "I" and the other first-person singular pronouns (1) when you are asked for a personal opinion or want to give one ("I think …" or "I believe …") or (2) when you have done the research or study and are reporting on it ("I found …" or "In my study, …"). When two people have collaborated, the proper personal pronoun would be "we" (and the other plural pronouns). Usually, in your formal assignments, it is better to keep personal pronouns to a minimum and to keep yourself in the background, unless you are asked for a personal opinion.

First-person pronouns may be used in some kinds of informal writing when you want to establish links between the writer and the reader. These pronouns help to create a warm, personal tone and to establish a relationship with the reader, as in the following example:

In our hospital, we frequently invite patients to "tell us what you think" in satisfaction surveys.

However, be sure that the informal tone is appropriate. One problem with pronouns is that readers cannot always be quite certain who is meant. Does "we" in the sentence above refer to the writer and the reader? the hospital administration? the unit manager? Consider the following sentence:

Nurses must take active roles in our society.

To whom does "our" refer: Canadian society? you and the instructor? Western society? nursing society? a specific association?

Finally, you also have to be careful of being too formal and avoiding the use of first-person pronouns altogether by referring to yourself as "the writer" or "this author." Such use can be confusing, as in this example:

These findings were reported by Baumgart (2019). This writer believes that ...

Does "this writer" refer to the writer of the assignment or to Baumgart?

Even the typeface (font) you use on your computer can help to set tone. Typical computer typefaces such as Courier and Times New Roman (similar to the type used for this book) are traditional and easy to read; they often are the default type used by your computer programs. Bold typefaces (**like this**) tend to be aggressive if used for complete sentences or paragraphs. Italic fonts (*like this*) are usually used in print to stress a word or phrase or to indicate a title. Some writers like to use an italic font in personal letters because it looks more like handwriting, but usually it is hard to read if used for long passages. Some of the newer typefaces are fashionable but hard to read except in headlines.

Another area where you need to consider tone is email messages. This is especially true today when many of you will be taking some courses online and will be communicating with your instructor and other students through email or a learning management system. Email is, in itself, an informal way of communicating. You probably have heard that using all capital letters in an email is considered "SHOUTING." If you use contractions (such as "I'm" instead of "I am"), sentence fragments (incomplete sentences), and emojis, you make your message even more informal. Informality probably is appropriate in messages to other students or to friends and relatives. However, informality might not be appreciated in communications with your instructors. For example, if you are communicating with an instructor in an email about an assignment, you need to consider how he or she would like to be approached. You could open the message with either of the following:

Hey, Mary - Assignment #1 is hairy! ;-) What exactly do you want? OR

Professor Smith - I am experiencing great difficulty in determining exactly what kind of reading I should be doing for Assignment 1. Do you wish us to use articles from research journals only; if so, how do we find these? And how many such readings would be appropriate?

Almost every instructor would consider the first example inappropriate. Example two certainly is more specific, although your instructor may have suggested that you could use a first name rather than "Professor." Chapter 5 contains more on email messages, but you always need to keep tone in mind.

See Box 1.3 for a quick summary of the SMART elements.

BOX 1.3   Thinking SMART for Student Papers

Source: In student assignments (essays, presentations), the source is *you* (or a group of students including you); evaluate your expertise in the subject and consider whether you need to provide supporting materials (references), what kind, and how many.

Message: This relates to the content of your paper—the topic and how you develop it.

Audience: This refers to the primary receiver of your written communication—for example, in a student paper, this is usually your instructor, although an instructor may sometimes ask you to write your assignment as if directed toward patients, health professional colleagues, or the public.

Route: A student paper is one route and differs from others (e.g., letter, email message, pamphlet, chart, personal journal, blog, media posting). Knowing the rules for student papers is essential.

Tone: The tone in a student paper would be formal.

POINTS TO REMEMBER

- The SMART elements of communication—Source * Message * Audience * Route * Tone—form a package deal that will help you with all your communications.

- Most problems that occur with your written assignments come back to a consideration of one (or more) of these elements. Although they interact with one another and you cannot separate them in the finished version, you do have to weigh each one carefully as you write.

❏ Once you get into the habit of examining your writing in the light of these five elements, you will improve your papers.

REFERENCES

American Psychological Association. (2010). *Publication manual of the American Psychological Association* (6th ed.). Washington, DC: Author.

Modern Language Association. (2016). *MLA handbook* (8th ed.). New York: Author.

Truss, L. (2004). *Eats, shoots & leaves: The zero tolerance approach to punctuation*. New York: Gotham Books/Penguin.

Turabian, K. L. (2018). *A manual for writers of research papers, theses, and dissertations: Chicago style for students and researchers* (9th ed.). Chicago: University of Chicago Press.

You are probably reading this text because you want to learn how to write more easily. You want to be able to write an excellent essay in one short sitting and avoid doing several drafts. Unfortunately, as dramatist Richard Sheridan, back in the 1700s, said: "Easy writing's curst hard reading" (as cited in Bartlett, 1940, p. 279). As almost every professional writer will tell you, writing well is hard work. Good writers usually go through several drafts so that readers can appreciate the results. However, if you understand the *process* involved in preparing written communications, you will save time and effort and produce a better finished paper.

One of the biggest problems for every writer is getting started. Sometimes the problem is simply procrastination; you plan to write but keep putting it off until you are "organized." So you tidy the desk, make coffee, feed the goldfish, straighten the bookshelf, mow the lawn, clean the fireplace, water the plants—and put off writing until the last possible moment (usually the evening before the paper is due). Recognize that written assignments are important and deserve your attention. Furthermore, when you start work on your assignment, devote yourself to it. Let your phone ring or go to voicemail; turn off the notification on your email and texts. Avoid multitasking and focus on the assignment.

So how should you begin to write a formal paper? You break down the big job into a series of separate steps, and then you take the first one—just as you would eat a dinosaur—one bite at a time. Good writers go through several logical steps, and it may be helpful for you to devote some time to each of them. A good way to start is to use the acronym PROCESS, which stands for **P**lan, **R**esearch, **O**rganize, **C**reate, **E**dit, **S**hine, and **S**ubmit. Figure 2.1 shows this as a ladder with various rungs that you must climb as you write your papers. Most student writers try to leap onto the ladder at the fourth rung; they plan just to sit down and write the assignment. You will have much greater success with your assignments if you deliberately spend some time on the ground and the first two rungs. Furthermore, you should make some specific deadlines for yourself. Do this as early as possible in the course. Read through your course syllabus and note the due dates

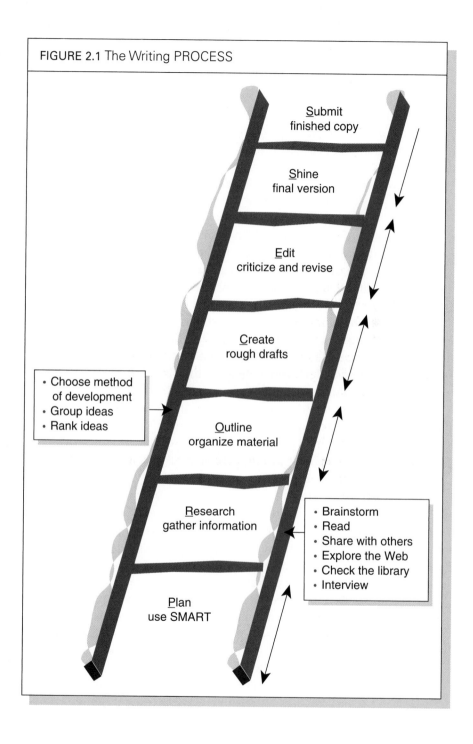

FIGURE 2.1 The Writing PROCESS

Submit
finished copy

Shine
final version

Edit
criticize and revise

Create
rough drafts

Outline
organize material

• Choose method
  of development
• Group ideas
• Rank ideas

Research
gather information

• Brainstorm
• Read
• Share with others
• Explore the Web
• Check the library
• Interview

Plan
use SMART

for assignments. Begin right away to think about the first assignment and continue to think about it as you read the first lessons or attend the first lectures. PROCESS helps you to manage your time effectively.

Spend the next few minutes examining the ladder diagram. The arrows indicate that you may need to go back and forth. For example, you may plan to write on a certain topic, but when you begin to look for information, you find that nothing is available. So you may need to step back and think about a new topic. Or, when you begin to organize your paper, you find that you need to go back and do further reading or thinking. An excellent idea is to note the date your assignment is due and then set a specific deadline for the first step.

Managing your time efficiently at this point is a key to successful academic writing. If you start writing your papers just when deadlines are looming, or if you start planning early and then get distracted, you need to improve your time management. Set interim deadlines for yourself, write these into your datebook, and then work on them! If you need more on time management, numerous helpful websites can help you identify your personal challenges (e.g., google "time management"). Allowing adequate time to attend systematically to each element of SMART and PROCESS will improve your writing dramatically. So let us use PROCESS to break down your assignment into steps.

PLAN (RUNG 1)

A planning step to take early in your program is to establish an effective and efficient space to do your writing. You may do your best creative thinking in a big, soft armchair, sipping coffee early in the morning before anyone else in the house is about. Or you may need to sit at a table in the library so that you can concentrate (and perhaps get away from noisy roommates or children). Or you may need to set up a desk in a corner at home. Remember that attending university or college and writing good papers is work! Give some thought to setting up a proper workplace.

You also need to know how to use and access computer programs that can help you to improve your writing skills. Take time to learn which dictionary your spell-checker uses (British or American) and what your spell-checker will or will not do. For example, a spell-checker probably will not pick up typos. If you type "I was a chemistry mayor at the University of Toronto," the spell-checker may not point out that the word intended was "major."

Computer programs also have a grammar checker—which may seem like a foe or friend. Many students will not use it because, when they try to check a long document, the grammar checker stops at almost every phrase and queries whether it should be fixed. It may then take you hours to identify which corrections are necessary. However, if you use the grammar checker on small portions of your writing, especially at first, it can be a valuable tool for improving your grammar. Grammar checkers also give you information about the "reading level" (e.g., Grade 8 or Grade 12 reading level) and about the "fog index" (e.g., multisyllable words, passive voice, long sentences) that makes it difficult for readers to find your point. If your computer program offers these features, learn how to use them.

You also need to begin to develop a way to have easy access to information—whether hardcopy or electronic—and to use information from all your courses. Libraries with multiple databases and vast digital collections of books and other resources make an overwhelming amount of content available. Skill is needed, however, to locate, select, evaluate, and organize a collection for use in your current and future assignments. This is called curation. As an effective curator, you locate the most authoritative, appropriate, complete, and current information and determine a strategy for storing it so that you can find what you need when you need it. Software programs (e.g., EndNote and RefWorks) are helpful in formatting references you may use throughout your program so that you can search your own collection of resources. You may even want to begin a working bibliography. It may also be helpful to keep a bookshelf, or file drawers or boxes, accessible to contain hardcopy information (or electronic folders for online resources).

Now for some specific information related to the planning step for each assignment. In many assignments, especially in your first year, your instructor will determine the topic for you. In some assignments, you may choose your own topic. In either case, you need to sit and think before you sit and write! You even need to determine a possible topic before you begin to gather information. If you spend a few minutes thinking about your assignment and sorting out in your mind the SMART elements of communication (Source * Message * Audience * Route * Tone) as they apply to the assignment, you will be much further ahead. If you can choose your own topic, choose it carefully. Although it is a good idea to select a topic that you (source) like, you also need to select one that fits with the other four elements. Are you knowledgeable about the topic, or will you have to do a great deal of background reading? Is the topic one that the instructor (audience) asked for or just one on which you want to write? Think about your proposed topic (message) carefully. Is it too big to be covered in a paper of 10 pages or 2000 words? If so, perhaps you should consider doing only one aspect of that topic. Is there enough information if you are asked to write a paper of 12 pages or 3000 words? Can you get information on this topic? Is this topic suitable for the type of assignment (route) you are asked to submit (book review, essay, personal journal, patient interview)? You may need to take the next step and do some preliminary library research (see Chapter 3) before you can tell whether your proposed topic is feasible.

Think first about the audience (your instructor). Read the information about the assignment carefully. What has your instructor specifically asked for in the assignment? What has he or she told you about the topic in class? What references have been suggested in your course outline or in class as being pertinent to the topic? Think about the instructor's purpose in giving the assignment. Is the purpose to see if you understand a point that was made in class or in some of the readings? Are you expected to answer a question in the paper, and is that answer to be based on reading or on personal experience or both? If you are to determine your own topic, ask yourself if your instructor is likely to be knowledgeable about that subject or whether you are more expert and will need to provide explanations.

This thinking or planning stage takes a bit of time, but it has two positive aspects. First, you can do it almost anywhere (e.g., riding home on the bus, waiting in the cafeteria for a friend). Second, it gets you started. And, if you like to be creative, it can be a highly stimulating time.

RESEARCH (RUNG 2)

After thinking about the five SMART elements, you will probably need to do some preliminary research before you can decide on your topic and plan for the next steps. For your first assignments, usually this means reading what experts have said about the topic. In most courses, your instructors will give you lists of readings, and some of them will likely apply. However, you should do additional research—and carefully consider the quality and reliability of the information you assemble.

You may find it helpful to talk to others about the topic. Conversing informally over coffee with fellow students or visiting online chat rooms or forums for your course may give you some ideas. Doing research in the digital age demands vigilance, however, because not all information is appropriate for professional use. Some may be completely inaccurate. Remember, you do not have to use ideas if they do not fit with what you, the source, want to say. You might discuss the subject over dinner with non-nursing friends or family; you might be surprised to find that family members can suggest some good ideas! But likely, you will need to supplement these ideas with expert views.

You are required to develop information literacy skills to locate, retrieve, sort through, store, and use quality information successfully. As some information is available only online, you also need digital and technical literacy skills. You need to understand how to use various electronic devices, search engines, and networks (including cloud computing). You should apply critical thinking to locate, evaluate, and select useful information from many media resources. As well, you should begin to assemble a list of materials you review that may remain with you (stored electronically) throughout your career (or at least as long as you are a student) because material for one course frequently will apply in another.

As you select information during your research, you must be mindful of rules for use of copyrighted materials. You need to know a great deal about attribution, or how to correctly acknowledge the source of your material. Copyright rules apply both to print resources and to multimedia elements, such as a clip from a newscast used during a presentation. Whole books have been written on copyright rules, and some lawyers earn their living on this subject, but you need a general awareness of how to deal with this or risk being accused of plagiarism. We go into this in more detail in Chapter 3.

You also need to consider whether you are using an original document (a "primary resource") or someone else's interpretation of the original document (a "secondary resource"). Research reports and information from recognized experts are the best resources for your assignments and they are less likely to contain misinterpretations or conjecture. If at all possible, you should try to review the primary resource to be certain that your secondary resource has accurately interpreted the information. Try Exercise 2.1 to practice your skill with information literacy.

Exercise 2.1 Searching for Resources

Read the following bits of information that you could use in a paper about helping older adult residents in an extended care facility get to sleep. The facility's physician does not wish to order sedatives (such as phenobarbital, which may be habit-forming and lead to withdrawal symptoms if taken too often).

1. You remember your grandmother used to drink a cup of camomile tea at bedtime and recommended it highly. You also recall a Beatrix Potter story from your childhood, where Peter Rabbit was given a cup of camomile tea by his mother to help him sleep after he escaped from Mr. McGregor's garden. Indicate whether you believe you could use this data in your

article and whether the information would be reliable and credible. Are these primary or secondary resources if you use them in your assignment?

2. You have seen advertisements on television and an article in a health shop magazine for a nonprescription, non–habit-forming, over-the-counter medication called "Deeep-Sleeepz" (we made this one up) and you look it up on the Internet. You find a website from the manufacturer that describes its virtues and tells you it is available inexpensively in a local health food shop, and you also locate two articles from natural remedy magazines that recommended it for their readers. You record the citation information for the articles and the information about the website. Are these primary or secondary resources and would you use them in your assignment?

3. You decide to ask three residents in the extended care facility if they have a favourite remedy they have used over the years to help them sleep and cite this information as personal communications. Is this information a primary or secondary resource and would you use it in your assignment?

4. You have read several articles about benefits of exercise in promoting healthy sleep and you yourself jog every evening because you find it helps you sleep. You search the professional journals and find several articles that support regular exercise as an aid to sleep. You are thinking of recommending an age-appropriate exercise program, such as a walking tour of the facility (outside, weather permitting) for residents to attend every evening before they go to their rooms. Then a classmate tells you that exercising before bed is not good because it increases the heart rate and releases epinephrine. In checking this out you find a reference on the WebMD website, which purportedly is a reputable resource; it reported on a study by the National Sleep Foundation that polled 1,000 participants and found that 83% of people do have better quality sleep when they exercise and that only 3% of people were adversely affected by exercising before bed (DiChiara, 2018). Are these all primary or secondary resources, and would you use them in your assignment?

COMMENTS ON EXERCISE 2.1 SEARCHING FOR RESOURCES

Remember that your answers to all of these exercises should reflect the SMART elements! You as the source, your message, the audience for it (mainly your instructor), other research you may do, and the tone of the article will be the guiding principles on whether you use any or all of the above—and how much other research you need to do. Given these comments as a basis, we offer a few additional observations on each of the above.

1. If you are going to discuss natural remedies for helping residents get to sleep in your assignment, you probably could use both examples in an anecdotal way if you have room. You could provide the information about your grandmother as an example and you would not need to indicate that it was a "personal communication" (described in Chapter 3). You also could refer to the Beatrix Potter story within the narrative as an item of general knowledge without a specific citation (as we did within the question). However, we would recommend that you also search for information from resources that are more reputable for health professionals. For example, the website of the Mayo Clinic (https://www.mayoclinic.org), a credible site for general health information for the public, notes camomile is generally safe for short-term use but can increase risk of bleeding for those on prescribed blood-thinning drugs and may cause allergic reactions. You also should check professional websites. The U.S. Food and Drug Administration (FDA) website (https://www.fda.gov) is credible for general information about drugs, and Health Canada (https://www.canada.ca/en/health-canada/services/drugs-health-products) also has a reliable site, but it is not as easy to search. The *Compendium of Pharmaceuticals and Specialties* (CPS) (Canadian Pharmacy Association, 2015), which you likely can access online through your college, university, or agency, is the most complete, unbiased, and accurate site.

2. Health professionals are generally leery about information put out by advertisers and manufacturers of over-the-counter medications as the information may exaggerate their claims and the quality of research. So you should look for information that might be more accepted by health professionals (including your instructor). If you did decide to use it, the manufacturer's website could be considered a primary resource (although perhaps a dubious one). The articles in the health remedy magazines would likely be considered secondary resources but may not be considered as good quality by your audience (your instructor), depending on whether the authors qualify as experts.

3. Here you are doing your own primary research (albeit with a tiny sample); doing your own research is good, but you can run into some pitfalls—mainly because universities and colleges have rules about the ethics of interviewing patients. You would definitely need to describe this in your assignment as an "informal" interview and report on the answers in a general way. You would not use the names of the residents nor cite any of the interviews as personal communications. Such initiative, however, would indicate you are thinking independently in

gathering information for the assignment. As well, the responses might be enlightening to you and might be great ice-breakers for conversations with your patients, as long as you keep the discussion general. You might want to check with your instructor about his or her thoughts on this before you interview patients or include this information.

4. You probably can find several articles that support regular exercise as an aid to sleep—but read them carefully. The DiChiara article is from a reputable website and could be considered a quality resource if you were writing the article about healthy adults; unfortunately, it does not make any mention of ages and the statistics therefore may not apply to senior residents in your facility. If you used the article for an assignment on healthy adults, it could be considered a secondary resource that cites a primary reference.

OUTLINE (RUNG 3)

The next step on the ladder is to organize your information into an intelligent outline, or plan for communication. You may find it helpful to brainstorm. Jot down all the ideas that pop into your head that you may want to develop in the assignment; do this briefly, using only two or three words for each. You could do this as a list or as a "mind map" in which you put the central idea in the middle of a page and then group other ideas around it. When a sub-idea sparks other ideas, you group them around the sub-idea. Some instructors refer to this as "clustering." This mind mapping is especially helpful if you are working on assignments with a partner or with a group. Remember, there are no bad ideas; silly suggestions may trigger an important concept or stimulate your co-authors. If not, you can throw it out. During the brainstorming stage, jot down as many ideas as possible—you can never have too many ideas during brainstorming.

For example, suppose your instructor suggests general topics for a written assignment, such as "Images of a health professional" or "Information sharing among health professionals" or "Evidence-based practice." You decide to jot down ideas about images of a health professional. You have some recommended materials on the topic, and these should get you started as shown in Exercise 2.2.

Exercise 2.2 Brainstorming

Try a 5-minute brainstorming session and create a map for a 10-page college-level paper on the topic "Pros and Cons of Wearing Uniforms." In addition to the topic (message), you also need to consider the other SMART elements right at the start. You (source) may have some definite opinions on this topic; would it be appropriate to the audience (your instructor) to include examples of why you believe as you do? Do you want to include photographs or illustrations in the paper (your route)? Do you want to be casual and humourous, using cartoons or funny stories, or would this not be an appropriate tone? The first map likely will reflect some of the questions that arise in your own mind.

COMMENTS ON EXERCISE 2.2 BRAINSTORMING

As you think about the topic for a few minutes, other questions may arise about the message, such as the following:

- "Do all health professionals wear uniforms? When and why do they wear them?"
- "Why did nurses, for example, wear standard uniforms that represented their schools of nursing? Why did they wear caps? Why did they stop wearing standard uniforms—and when?" Perhaps you could even make a big circle around these points and list them as "History of Uniforms in Nursing."
- "Does wearing a uniform take away your individuality?"
- "Does a uniform contribute to (or take away from) a professional image?"
- "Should uniforms be white or coloured—and why?"
- "What do patients think about uniforms?"
- "Should the uniform be appropriate for the setting in which you are working?"
- "Should uniforms reflect departments, such as operating room, pediatric unit, emergency department, pharmacy, rehabilitation, or occupational therapy?"

You, and various people you may talk to, including other students, graduates, and patients, may raise other points. But you also need to think about the course for which this paper is required: Did you discuss "professionalism" in your classes, and were uniforms mentioned in the discussion? Did any of your assigned readings raise the topic of uniforms? Are uniforms mentioned in your textbook readings? Will your instructor (audience) expect you to refer to some of these or to some other points?

In the early mapping, you should write down as many ideas as you can think of, whether pros or cons. Then, if you have strong opinions one way or the other, you may want to make your paper reflect these and conclude that some health professionals should wear a standard uniform in certain settings. Refer to the map in Figure 2.2 for ideas about how a nurse might make a map on this subject.

As you think about your map over the next few days, you may realize that you need to do some research to see what reputable and trustworthy

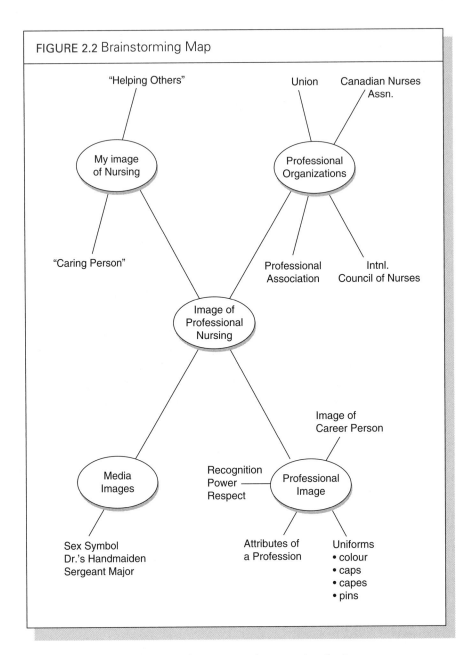

FIGURE 2.2 Brainstorming Map

"Helping Others"

Union   Canadian Nurses
              Assn.

My image
of Nursing

Professional
Organizations

"Caring Person"

Professional   Intnl.
Association   Council of Nurses

Image of
Professional
Nursing

Image of
Career Person

Media
Images

Recognition
Power
Respect

Professional
Image

Sex Symbol
Dr.'s Handmaiden
Sergeant Major

Attributes of
a Profession

Uniforms
• colour
• caps
• capes
• pins

resources have said about uniforms. You also may decide that you want to talk even more to others. You may want to see if there have been patient satisfaction surveys or other research completed on clients' views about the areas in which you do your clinical practice. Or you may want to ask all the graduates on the unit for their opinions (if you can find time to do this during your clinical session). You may also want to ask further questions of your instructor and classmates, either in class or online.

Remember that the map does not need to be neat and tidy; it represents a brainstorming session, and its purpose is to get you to start thinking. Jot down one or two words to reference any ideas that come to mind, even if you think they may not be relevant later; for example, you might want to write the word "shoes" to remind yourself later to consider whether standard shoes are part of a uniform. You may want to write the word "cost" to remind you to think about whether standard uniforms would be more or less expensive. You may want to write the word "supplier" to remind you to think about whether the hospital or agency would supply uniforms (perhaps at a reduced rate).

Once you have come up with all the ideas that you want to put into your assignment, you need to organize them into some sort of order—you need an outline. Remember the essay outline you learned about in elementary school? Your first teachers urged you to organize your papers into *three* main parts. This is still a good idea, although it will not work for all topics. Some topics need two parts, whereas some need four or more parts. The rationale behind this division into main parts, however, is that readers will be able to follow your thoughts. Keeping the main divisions to a manageable number (such as three) helps readers to grasp your ideas readily and to remember them easily. You may cover more than three ideas within a paper, but some of them will be organized as subparts of one of the three main ideas. See Box 2.1.

BOX 2.1 Outline

I.   Introduction
II. Body
     A. First main idea
         1 Sub-idea to main idea
         2 Sub-idea to main idea
             a. Sub–sub-idea
             b. Sub–sub-idea
     B. Second main idea
         (and sub-ideas organized as in A)
     C. Third main idea
         (and sub-ideas organized as in A)
III. Conclusion

In the outlining stage, you should consider the length of the final paper. Almost all instructors specify length. Some instructors take off marks if a student writes a paper that is longer or shorter than specified. If at this point—*before* you begin to write—you consider the overall length, you can focus on the most important ideas and group the less important ideas so that you cover the greatest amount of information without putting too much emphasis on one point. You can decide to omit some details, or you can select one example to stand for several others. If you are conscious of length right from the beginning, you will not have to spend hours later trying to shorten a lengthy draft. As well, you will be less likely to ramble once you begin to write.

You also help your readers to understand your message by telling them in the introduction just what you are going to cover in the main part of the paper. And in the concluding section, you sum up your ideas briefly to remind the reader what was covered. In the journalistic world, this organizational pattern is summed up this way:

- Tell them what you are going to tell them.
- Tell them.
- Tell them what you have told them.

This framework may sound rather simplistic, but you can still be creative within it. Remember that an assignment is not a mystery novel in which you save your point until the end of the book. Making your point clearly in the introduction will certainly help your instructor understand what you are doing with your paper—and will likely pay off in marks!

You may want to finish the outline stage by jotting down several ideas for a title; doing so helps you to define your idea. Let your mind go; be creative. Try to summarize the main idea in one or two sentences or in those famous "25 words or less." If you start early enough, you can take a few minutes a day for several days in this phase. And you can do it anywhere, such as while driving to work or washing the car. Just be sure that you record the ideas for later use. Try Exercise 2.3 to practice outlining.

Exercise 2.3 Outlining

Look at the Brainstorming Map that was done in Exercise 2.2. Drawing on the ideas shown in this map (which you will augment by research), take a few minutes to prepare the beginnings of an outline—and then come back and review the following comments.

COMMENTS ON EXERCISE 2.3 OUTLINING

If you are a nurse, you may decide to limit your focus on the assigned subject of "Pros and Cons of Wearing Uniforms," and it might look something like this:

Working Title: "The Professional Image of Nurses Today"

I. Introduction

A general statement that the image of health professionals, including nurses, has changed and continues to change and is influenced by interpretations by the public, media, profession, and individual professional

II. Body of Paper

  A. Past images of nursing

    1. Old-fashioned images of nurses: starched uniforms, caps, capes; doctor's handmaiden; sex symbol; martinet

    2. Development of a profession

      • Graduate nurses, registered nurses, professional organizations (local, provincial, national, international)

      • Better education and changes for entry to practice

    3. Were these images accurate?

  B. Present images of nursing

    1. How does the public (and media) envision nurses today?

    2. How do nurses themselves envision "the nurse" (are there stereotypical images?)

    3. "Career" versus "job"

    4. Influence of unions

  C. Future images of nursing

    1. Will there be a "general image" in the future? Does there need to be a separate and distinct image? Will there be more than one image?

    2. ???

III. Summary

Statement relating the three sections back to the opening introduction and showing that the various images of nurses from the past and present will also affect the image of nurses in the future. Try to end with a memorable statement or even a quotation.

Note that this is only a beginning outline. As you do more reading and more research into the image of professional nurses (past, present, and future), the outline may change.

Alternatively, your map and its groupings may suggest that your paper would be divided into three parts: (1) Pros, (2) Cons, and (3) Recommendations. Do you want to conclude with a recommendation for one side or the other or merely provide a balanced viewpoint? Or you may decide that you want to make an outline for the body of your paper that deals with (1) Historical Background on Uniforms, (2) The Case Against Uniforms, (3) The Case for Uniforms. (Remember, you will also have a short introductory section and a short concluding section.)

CREATE (RUNG 4)

If you spend time on the three early rungs, then you should be able to write your first drafts for papers much more quickly than you have in the past. However, you should still plan on having to make at least one rough draft. Most professional writers say they need at least three. This does not necessarily mean that you completely retype your draft word for word each time. What you do is create a "working draft" that you can go over several times. Although with computers you can alter your original draft quickly, you may still want to save an earlier version in case you decide later that an earlier draft contains something you now need.

Ideally, you should create the first working copy quickly. A first draft should be creative; you concentrate on developing the main body of the message. From your brainstorming and outlining sessions, you already know the main points of your message, and you will have organized them to make your message clear and strong, keeping your audience in mind. You should be able to pick up words and phrases directly from your brainstorming page and outline and incorporate them into the first draft.

Probably you will need to use one paragraph to develop each of the ideas that you jotted down during your brainstorming session. Usually, a paragraph deals with one main idea, which is introduced in the first sentence (also called the topic sentence). This is followed by two or three (and occasionally more) sentences that develop the idea. The paragraph then frequently ends with a sentence that sums up the idea (called the concluding sentence). Note that this is similar to the way you develop the paper as a whole. Beware of paragraphs that are too long and too complex. Some instructors complain that students have paragraphs that go on for several pages.

You may still find it hard to begin writing at this point. The best way is merely to get some sentences down. Simply writing half a page or more gets you started. You may eventually scrap it, but you have started. Some instructors, especially during first-year courses, try to help students overcome a writing block by giving short assignments designed to help you improve both your writing and your thinking skills. These assignments often are described as "writing-to-learn" projects and are designed to help students acquire and interpret (for themselves as well as for others) the complex knowledge base needed. Such projects help students to clarify theoretical points or to reflect on ways that personal experiences ("lived experiences") can be applied; they are intended to help students develop conceptual approaches and thinking patterns that will be helpful in practice settings.

Such projects often involve "free writing" and "quick writing." Free writing often is assigned at the beginning of a class. Students spend about five minutes writing about their feelings (e.g., feelings after the first visit to a clinical placement or after the death of a patient), or about concerns or issues involving the student body (e.g., thoughts about a proposed student strike to protest a fee hike), or about a previous class or assignment (e.g., summaries of articles assigned as reading). For most of these "quick-write" assignments, instructors are concerned only with your ability to identify the main points or concepts (message) and are not as interested in grammar, spelling, punctuation, sentence and paragraph construction, and presentation (matters of route). However, these instructors may also use these writing-to-learn assignments to provide feedback about writing skills. Because these papers usually are short, an instructor takes time to identify writing-skill problems as well as to assess conceptualization skills.

Many instructors ask students to keep a daily (or weekly) log or journal in which they describe their feelings, summarize their classroom or clinical learning, or raise issues for discussion in class. This is often referred to as "journalling." These assignments are usually informal writings that you keep for your own personal use—although in this case you allow your instructor, and maybe your classmates, to share your thoughts. The principle behind these assignments is to get you to use words to capture ideas. And because you are choosing words to express your own thoughts, feelings, opinions, impressions, beliefs, emotions, or concerns, you do it without having to turn to the writings of others. This gives you practice with thinking in words and putting these on paper so others can see your views and understand them. These assignments are often done to encourage reflection. Reflection helps you to delve more deeply into your thoughts so that you can express them clearly. For, as the English poet George Gordon, Lord Byron (as cited in Colombo, 1974, p. 91), wrote in the early 1800s:

> ... words are things, and a small drop of ink,
> Falling like dew, upon a thought, produces
> That which makes thousands, perhaps millions think.

You often learn from these small exercises that you do have good writing skills and that you do have thoughts that are meaningful and worth sharing. Some instructors ask students to write poetry as one way of getting in touch with their feelings through the experience of capturing them in words—and some of these poems are real gems.

Usually, your instructor will tell you how the journal or the quick-writes should be set up (the rules of the route), such as double-spaced in a Word document or in a private blog. For these writing-to-learn projects, you still need to think SMART and to go through the steps that make up the writing PROCESS, even though you must do it more quickly than with a longer paper.

You can practise free writing or quick writing on your own. Writing things down helps you to understand theoretical points or reflect on ways personal experiences can be applied. Such practice helps you to develop conceptual approaches and thinking patterns that will also be helpful in practice settings.

Once you are caught up in the act of the writing, your thoughts will become more organized. Many writers like to complete the body of the paper first and then turn to the introduction and conclusion. Other writers like to write the introduction first because it helps them to clarify exactly what they want to say and the order in which to say it. Either way, you want to keep the introductory and concluding sections short, especially during the first draft. You can come back to them during the next steps when you edit and revise.

Writing the first draft is not the time to worry about spelling or grammar; you can fix these errors later. But do be aware when you are using materials—either direct quotes or paraphrases—from someone else. Have a system for easily locating these resources later, but at this point do not worry about getting the reference information down in detail; keep this chore for the time you are doing your reference list.

At this point, you should be trying to put the message into your own words, showing that you truly understand it. Be creative and remember that this is merely the *beginning* of the paper; knowing that this version does not have to be perfect helps you to let your ideas flow. Visualize your instructor reading it. See your paper as a kind of long, informative letter with a specific message from you. Focus on getting your whole message across.

Once you have your first draft finished, try to leave it and take a break. If you can leave it overnight and edit the next day, you will likely be able to read the paper and easily spot areas that need to be worked on further. If you are organized enough to do the first draft several days in advance, then you will even have time to do a bit more research if necessary.

When you come back to your first draft, continue at first to concentrate on the message rather than on details of spelling and grammar. Ask yourself if you got the main point across clearly so that any reader could understand it. Are the subordinate points obvious so that the reader can follow them clearly? You may want to add more in one section, elaborate some point, or give an example to make your point clearly. All good writers have revised their drafts, from Charles Dickens to Ernest Hemingway to J. K. Rowling.

Keep considering the length as you work. On a computer, you can quickly find a word count. Eventually, you will achieve a copy that contains the message you are satisfied with—or, more likely, you will run short of time! Either way, you still need to go over the draft version at least once more—and that is Rung 5.

EDIT (RUNG 5)

During the final reviews of the draft, you stop creating the message and start to concentrate on critiquing and improving the writing. Even minor errors can be enormously distracting to readers—and thus destroy your credibility and bring your abilities as a writer or researcher into question. Now is the time to look at vocabulary, grammar, punctuation, and spelling. Consider the tone of the essay. Is it too formal? Have you used an appropriate vocabulary for a college-level paper? Have you used professional language ("abdomen" rather than "tummy"; "intestine" rather than "gut")? Have you borrowed jargon from the readings without understanding it? Are your words too pretentious? A general rule is that clear, simple, appropriate words convey your message the best. Use your critical faculties.

Stop looking at what you want to say and concentrate on saying it well and clearly. You need to be sure you have not made errors in grammar or word usage, and that your spelling is consistent. Your computer will aid you with grammar and usage. You may want to turn this function off while you are writing the first drafts, but at this point you may want to use it. You may find it more useful just to highlight one page at a time, rather than face a sea of errors marked throughout the whole paper. Such errors are fine in the first drafts. If you begin using your computer tools early in your writing career, and use them in small doses, they will act as a "computer tutor" and help you gradually improve your writing skills.

When you begin to revise, concentrate especially on creating good, clear writing in the introductory and concluding sections of the paper. These sections are vital because they make the most impact on readers. You want to start with strong, clearly stated, and, if possible, memorable sentences.

And you want to end your message by clearly reviewing what you tried to achieve in the body of the paper. The words of your final paragraph will leave a lasting impression on your instructor as he or she works out your mark. So consider these sections carefully. Many great authors suggest that you spend as much time on the first and the last paragraphs as you do on the rest of the paper!

When you edit your paper, concentrate on the "flow" of ideas and make certain that your message is obvious to the audience. Instructors frequently stress to us that students fail to understand this point. You may find some instructors will indicate "lack of flow" in feedback on your paper. "Flow" refers to logical streaming of ideas from beginning to end. Often you will have good ideas, but if you do not link them in a clear, logical order, readers will find it difficult to follow your reasoning.

Clear flow is helped by little "road signs" that you put into your paper, such as "First, I want to …," and then, later in the paper, you write another marker, such as "Second, I propose to …." Other such markers, which often come at the beginning of new paragraphs, are:

> "Next, …"
> "On the other hand, …" (Just be careful you do not have more than two hands!)
> "In contrast to the idea discussed in the paragraphs above, …"

These road markers, often described in writing textbooks as "transitions" or as "linking words or phrases," help the reader to follow your argument.

A useful hint at this stage is to read the paper aloud to yourself, listening to the words and grammar rather than to the message. Does the sentence sound right, or can it be misinterpreted? Consider these newspaper headlines that slipped by editors:

> "Drunken Drivers Paid $1,000 Last Week"
> "Local High School Dropouts Cut in Half"
> "Miners Refuse to Work after Death"

Watch for sentences that are too long to read comfortably. Do you get lost halfway through a sentence? Do you fail to understand what a pronoun refers to? If you have trouble, think how difficult it will be for your instructor or other readers.

You might find it helpful to get someone else to read your work. Print out a copy and look at it yourself as well. You will find an amazing number of points that slipped by you on the computer screen but show up on the hard copy. If the reader wants to make comments on a computer version, suggest he or she use a different colour or font so that it will stand out or use one of the editing tools that comes with your computer program (e.g., Track Changes or comment boxes). Try to find someone who is helpful but not overly critical; all writers are vulnerable when they give a draft to someone to review. The person need not be an expert on the content, but pick someone who can learn from reading your paper—and he or she will learn from it only if it is clearly written. You want a friend who will offer some praise and positive feedback as well as some useful critical comments. Remember, too, that you do not have to accept and use all the criticisms.

Chapter 4 gives more detail on common errors in writing and on other points to look for when you are editing the final draft. Try Exercise 2.4 now to test your knowledge of grammar.

Exercise 2.4 Grammar, Usage, Spelling, and Punctuation

This short paragraph contains errors in grammar, usage, spelling, and punctuation. See how many you can spot and correct.

In order to efficiently apply for most senior positions, resumes should be used. Potential applicants often seek advise from communication experts in designing their résumés, however some of the suggestions from these consultants are a bit flamboyant and they are unsuited to conservative healthcare institutions. All recommendations should be weighed carefully. Noone should accept poor council which may effect their futures.

COMMENTS ON EXERCISE 2.4 GRAMMAR, USAGE, SPELLING, AND PUNCTUATION

- Change *In order to efficiently apply* to *To apply* (unnecessary words).
- Delete *most* (unnecessary).
- Be consistent in spelling throughout the paper; note that the spelling of resumes in the next sentence is résumés.
- Change resumes to résumés (the spelling recommended in your style guide).
- Change *résumés should be used* to *applicants should use résumés* (résumés do not apply for senior positions—applicants do; poor sentence and passive voice).

- Change *Potential applicants* to *Many job hunters* (clarity; shorter words; prevents repetition of applicants in the rewritten version).
- Change *advise* to *advice* (either a misused word or a typing error).
- Change *in designing their résumés* to *about résumé design* (ambiguous pronoun reference; *their* could refer to experts or to applicants).
- Change the comma to a semicolon before *however* and insert a comma after *however* (original is a "run-on sentence"; alternative: change the comma to a period and start the next sentence with *However* and a comma).
- Delete *of the* (unnecessary).
- Change *consultents* to *consultants* (either a spelling mistake or a typing error; tighten the sentence by removing *a bit*, a lazy and vague modifier, and then reword the latter part of the sentence both to remove the pronoun *they*, which could refer to *consultants*, and to reduce the length of the sentence).
- Change *All recommendations should be weighed carefully* to *Weigh recommendations carefully* (removes passive voice).
- Change *Noone* to *No one* (either a spelling mistake or a typing error).
- Change *council* to *counsel* (misuse of word).
- Change *which* to *that* (misuse of word).
- Change *effect* to *affect* (misuse of word).
- Change *their futures* to *his or her future* (lack of agreement; pronoun[s] must agree in number with *No one*; alternative: change *their futures* to *one's future*).

The following is the revised, polished version (47 words compared with 61 words in the original; average number of words per sentence is 12 compared with 15.5 in the original; one long sentence with 22 words compared with one long sentence with 32 words in the original):

> To apply for senior positions, applicants should use résumés. Many job hunters seek advice from communication experts about résumé design; however, suggestions from some consultants may be unsuitable for healthcare professionals. Weigh recommendations carefully. No one should accept poor counsel that may affect his or her future.

SHINE (RUNG 6)

Now is the time for you to "shine" or polish your work. Minor errors, such as typos, tarnish the image you want to present. Start to concentrate on following the style guide required in your program. As you prepare the final copy, look at the general format, such as headings, spacing, table of contents, size of type, and so on. These are all points related to route, and we go into these points in more detail for first-year student papers in Appendix A. If you are in a more senior year, you probably need access to a style manual that spells out the rules of the route in detail. Or, if you are looking at rules for other presentations (e.g., business letters, electronic communications, résumés, business reports), you should review Chapter 5. Also consider your quotations, citations, references, and bibliographies (if these are needed), which are addressed in Chapter 3.

You need to turn in a final version that is clean and easy to read. Just as you would not appear for a job interview in dirty, ragged gardening clothes, so must your paper appear in a suitable form. Unless the instructor has advised otherwise, you probably will submit your paper electronically, but it still must follow the general rules for print papers. Be aware that there may be difficulties with electronic submissions; some seem to disappear into cyberspace, so be sure you keep a backup copy. There is a possibility that some of your formatting (e.g., graphics, figures, fonts, colours) could be lost or distorted when you submit your paper electronically. To prevent this, you can convert your Microsoft Word file to a Portable Document Format (PDF); these files display your paper exactly as it was created. Ask your instructor if a PDF version is appropriate.

Generally speaking, you set up an electronic paper to resemble the hardcopy formats used in the past. You need to be sure that the default settings on your word processing program are those recommended in the style guide for your course. Standard margins are usually programmed into your word processor or computer, although you can change them. In the past, one-inch margins allowed instructors room to write notes and comments on the paper—and one-inch margins at the top, bottom, and left and right sides of the page are still generally recommended even though instructors now have options for providing electronic feedback (such as Track Changes, Google Docs, or other comment boxes). As always, your instructor's special requirements override all other style guidelines.

Double-space your essays even in electronic submissions; doing so makes them easier to read. Because your assignment is a finished product in itself and not a manuscript being submitted to a publisher, you may need to use single spacing for some parts of your paper. Some style manuals advise single spacing in tables, long quotations, and footnotes. Generally, you double space your references and bibliographies to make them easier to read, although some style manuals require single spacing. If so, you then double space between entries to make it easier for the reader.

Some class assignments do not follow rigidly the rules of style guides; for example, your instructor may ask you to submit a title page and table of contents. (Instructors often do this to see if you have been working from an outline!) You may choose to alter the spacing to improve the appearance. You can see what your overall page looks like by choosing from options in the "View" tab in Microsoft Word.

Page numbers are really helpful and are usually required in student essays. But again, style rules vary. Most style manuals recommend you number your pages in the top right-hand corner, using Arabic numbers in the same font as used in the body of your paper. Number the title page as well.

For long submissions, such as theses or dissertations, style manuals note preliminary pages may be given lower case Roman numerals (e.g., i, vii); Arabic numbering starts with a 1 on the first page of the main part. This usually is not done with short student assignments.

As a final step, you should read over the paper just once more before you turn it in. You may find a few typing errors (e.g., "works" instead of "words") that slipped by previous proofreading or were not picked up on the spell-checker. Or you may find a place where there was a small breakdown in the computer codes, which caused minor errors or typos in a few words or lines. See also Chapter 4 on common errors.

Exercise 2.5 gives you some ideas on how to shine your sentences.

Exercise 2.5 Shining Up the Final Copy

1. Delete extraneous words in the following sentences:
   - He is in the process of drawing up the nominations.
   - She intends to take action without further delay.

2. Polish the following poor sentences:
   - She did not think that it was unimportant to wear neat, professional dress.
   - The union was not unwilling to negotiate on the offer.
   - Well Known Hospital (WKH) will be responsible for the development and execution of a health promotion day designed to increase awareness in the local community about WKH's Wellness Clinic.

3. Think about the double meanings in the following sentences:
   - Yesterday, the police tied the suspect to the car used in the holdup.
   - New mothers find it much harder to manage when they have children.

COMMENTS ON EXERCISE 2.5 SHINING UP THE FINAL COPY

1. The following are shorter, clearer versions:
   - He is drawing up the nominations.
   - She intends to take action now.

2. The following are improved versions:
   - She thought that neat professional dress was important.
   - The union was willing to negotiate on the offer. (*This version avoids double negatives.*)

- Well Known Hospital will develop and carry out a health promotion day to inform the local community about its Wellness Clinic.
  OR
- Well Known Hospital will develop and carry out a health promotion day to help make the local community aware of its Wellness Clinic.

3. You could rewrite these sentences several ways, if you have time. These two humorous examples should remind you that sometimes you get too close to your work; although a sentence makes good sense to you, it may not make good sense to your readers.

SUBMIT (RUNG 7)

The final step in the writing process is to submit the paper. Instructors usually provide directions for submitting assignments, perhaps in the course syllabus; if not, then follow the departmental guidelines. Sometimes the route specified in the assignment dictates what you use (e.g., a blog entry for class discussion). Instructors often want or need a few extra things in a student paper that may not be specified in a style manual. For example, you may need to attach a cover letter (probably only one page); cover letters allow you to give additional details that may not be appropriate in a formal paper. For example, the letter might explain why the paper is late (or early, as the case may be). Or you might want to explain that your paper is directed to a specific audience, such as health care users or health care professionals. If you use a cover letter, it should be set up properly as a business letter (see Chapter 5).

Do submit your paper on time. Some instructors deduct marks (sometimes a large percentage of marks) for a late paper. One reason for doing so is that if other students manage to meet the deadline, you have an unfair advantage. Check the policies of your school. If you have a good reason for a delay, ask for an extension rather than submitting the paper late. Contact your instructor about an extension before the assignment due date. In an email message, provide sufficient detail regarding the reason you need an extension without going into long-winded explanations. Ask for a specific length of time for the extension, such as:

Professor Jones,
I am a student in your Health Studies 400 class. I am requesting a 24-hour extension to the due date for my term paper. I have had the flu this past week. Thank you for considering my request.
Sincerely, Sam Student

As a final step before you press send and submit your paper, go through the checklist for submission in Box 2.2.

You will find a sample student paper illustrating these points in Appendix A. Chapter 5 contains more information about specific routes other than the student paper.

BOX 2.2   Checklist for Submission (APA Style)

The following checklist reviews some of the points you need to keep in mind when shining up your paper for submission. If you are unclear about the meaning of some of these points, see Chapter 4.

- Check you are using the format required by your instructor.
- Set one-inch margins at the top, bottom, and left and right sides of all pages—or as recommended by your instructor. (These are usually the default margins.)
- Justify left margin but leave right margin unjustified ("ragged").
- Use a standard 12-point typeface with serifs, such as Times New Roman, CG Times, Courier, or Pica.
- Double-space lines in the main text (and in most other parts of the paper unless other spacings would improve appearance and readability).
- Number all pages in the top right-hand corner.
- Read the paper aloud: Is it easy to read, or do you stumble anywhere?
- Check the length of your sentences: Are there too many long ones?
- Do too many sentences start the same way? Look especially for sentences with weak openings such as "There are …" or "This is …" or "It was …."
- Check for improper use of first-person pronouns (*I, we, my, our, me, ours*).
- Have you used professional language or used jargon, slang, or clichés?
- Are too many sentences in the passive voice?
- Check the style of your title, headings, and subheadings.
- Check spellings of words about which you are not completely certain; if you use a spell-checker, learn how to use it but do not rely on it.

BOX 2.2   Checklist for Submission (APA Style)—Cont'd

- Check the use of capitals: Are they consistent? Do you have a reason for using the capital letters you used throughout your paper?
- Check the punctuation: Have you used a comma before the word *and* in a series of three or more items? Do you have too many commas? Are there quotation marks where they are needed? Have you used apostrophes appropriately? Are there too many dashes and exclamation points (which signal an informal tone)?
- Proofread the finished, printed copy through a final time; do not change your content but make any minor corrections.
- Keep a copy of your paper; even the best instructors occasionally misplace a paper.
- Always remember that your instructor's requirements outrank all other style guidelines.

POINTS TO REMEMBER

❏   The initial letters for each of the rungs or steps in Chapter 2 spell out PROCESS, which is an acronym for **P**lan, **R**esearch, **O**rganize, **C**reate, **E**dit, **S**hine, and **S**ubmit.

❏   Understanding PROCESS will help you write more effectively and efficiently. This acronym shows that good writing has several steps—and, if you want to write like a pro, the first three steps (PRO) are the most important.

❏   Students who have major problems with written communications tend to neglect these three basic steps of the ladder—and these early steps are usually the fun part of writing! They represent the time when you can let your imagination flow.

❏   The SMART elements of communication (Source * Message * Audience * Route * Tone) also are important as you proceed through the PROCESS steps.

❏   Getting started writing can be the hardest part. Just start brainstorming and jotting down ideas.

❑ Do not neglect to polish your work so your great ideas will shine through.

❑ Finally, remember that writing well is hard work for everybody, but when you take the time to finish the PROCESS you will be more successful.

REFERENCES

Bartlett, J. (1940). *Familiar quotations: A collection of passages, phrases, and proverbs traced to their sources in ancient and modern literature* (11th ed.). Boston, MA: Little, Brown.

Canadian Pharmacy Association. (2015). *The compendium of pharmaceuticals and specialties (CPS)*. Ottawa, ON: Author.

Colombo, J. R. (Ed.). (1974). *Colombo's Canadian quotations*. Edmonton, AB: Hurtig.

DiChiara, T. (2018). Can exercising at night hurt your sleep? Retrieved from https://www.webmd.com/sleep-disorders/features/can-exercising-at-night-hurt-your-sleep#1

As mentioned in Chapter 1, if you (source) are not an expert in a subject, you may need to substantiate information presented to the reader (audience), especially when your information (message) is controversial, theoretical, or new. Usually, you take information from a reliable resource, such as a research report or an expert, and include it to support your views. To do this properly in a formal paper (route), you need to know how to find new information and to acknowledge the material you use through in-text citations and references (the details of the full resource, usually listed at the end of the paper).

Citations, references, and bibliographies are essential components of college- and university-level papers. Furthermore, the need for reliable, well-chosen resources increases throughout your program. In your first-year papers, you may use only a few references, but you will use many more as you proceed through the program. As well, you must be able to use references on the job to guide evidence-based practice. If you decide to take a graduate degree, you will need to be familiar with several styles of citations, references, and bibliographies.

This chapter introduces you to ways of gathering information for your paper and helps you learn to use this material. It will also acquaint you further with some of the mysteries of style manuals and their roles in indicating resources used. The summary here will suffice for most papers in your early years, and your instructors will be offering you additional advice as you progress through your courses and your papers become more sophisticated.

This chapter also provides background information usually not included in style manuals and will:

- outline how to find information for your paper;
- explain how and why a citation is used;
- comment briefly on plagiarism;
- introduce you to different methods used for references (numerical style versus author–year style);
- describe what a complete citation includes; and
- identify three common reference errors that students often make in papers.

FINDING INFORMATION FOR YOUR PAPER

Assignments at the college and university level almost always require that you read widely, so you need to be familiar with the resources available. You likely will have been assigned one or two texts and numerous journal articles for the course, and they should form the basis for your reading. As well, you should check out the topic in texts for your other courses. Use the tables of contents and indexes to look for additional information about the subject. You may also find reference lists within these materials that direct you to even more information. In addition to your textbooks and lecture notes, there are many other places you can get information, including books and journals in libraries, Internet database searches, and personal communications (e.g., interviews, discussion boards, emails, and even tweets).

Library Research

You should start your search for information by looking at books and professional journals. You can do this in person or by using the campus online library catalogues; they allow you to search materials of interest to health professionals, such as databases of scholarly works, e-books, and video and audio materials. Do not neglect other libraries, such as the public library; you might also want to check local hospitals and other health agencies as some have excellent libraries of digital and print materials and allow staff and students to use them. Professional associations and unions also may have useful library resources, but make sure to ask if it costs money to use them.

Spend some time in your college or university library finding out what it offers (e.g., your library may have access agreements with expensive and hard-to-access facilities) and how to make effective use of its services. Libraries usually offer orientation courses at the beginning of each term; make time to participate in the orientation even if you think you are competent. Most libraries offer video tutorials on essential library skills, such as choosing productive keywords, searching databases, saving database histories, and using tools such as RefWorks or EndNote. Take time to view these as part of your orientation. Keywords are a quick and convenient way of searching. You use a carefully chosen word or words pertinent to your topic; this allows you to scan masses of resources looking for the most relevant material. Databases and computerized indexes for journal articles are often arranged by subject. Not all journals provide full articles over the Internet, so relying on e-journals may limit your findings. Most database options allow you to search "full-text only" articles. Sometimes you only have access to abstracts—but reviewing abstracts can be helpful because you get an overview of relevant published research.

You should look for articles on your subject in recent issues of professional journals in your discipline. The information in journal articles is often more up to date than that in books. The reading list for your course may identify a few such articles. However, spend some time looking for new articles on the subject; keeping abreast of the latest research always impresses an instructor. You can browse in e-journals relevant to your professional area—just be sure that these are peer-reviewed, reputable, credible journals (because not all journals are created equal). You will need to access peer-reviewed journals; these are journals in which each article has been through a review process by professionals who are experts in the area. Another way to find out about a journal's importance is to check the impact factor (IF) or journal impact factor (JIF); this reflects the relative quality and importance of the journal to professionals and is frequently mentioned in databases, in the journal, or on the journal's website.

It is important to recognize the differences between professional journals and lay magazines; both can provide important information for you, depending on your topic. For example, to find statistics on health professionals in the workforce or the health care system, you probably need to access materials from government agencies (such as the U.S. Department of Health and Human Services, Statistics Canada, or your professional associations and unions). Lay magazines and newspapers often have editorial comments on health care issues that can provide you with valuable input about political realities.

Several databases are of particular interest to students in health professions. One such database is CINAHL Plus; CINAHL stands for "Cumulative Index to Nursing and Allied Health Literature" and provides selected indexes, abstracts, and full-text articles from more than 4900 journals, including core health journals (e.g., *Cancer, The Lancet, Journal of Aging and Health,* and *RN,* to name just a few). The Plus means that this database also provides access to other resources such as dissertations, conference proceedings, standards of practice, audiovisuals, and more. The MEDLINE database focuses on medical and allied health journals; PsycINFO is an indexing service for psychology and allied disciplines. The Proquest Nursing and Allied Health Source database is useful to students from all health professions; it includes scholarly literature, clinical training videos, reference materials, dissertations, and systematic reviews. Academic Search Complete offers full-text journals related to the social sciences, humanities, science, technology, engineering, and mathematics, in addition to indexes and abstracts from almost 11,000 publications.

The databases will help you identify articles and resources through keywords. You also should check subject guides on your library's home page. A subject guide is an in-depth collection of the most useful links and authoritative resources within a subject area. Check back often for updates to subject guides.

Be certain that you make full and accurate notes about the materials you review, including who wrote the material, its proper title, and the place you found it. You often can copy the abstract or even the complete article from the online resources and save it in your reference files. Copying material when you find it may save you hours of work later, but make sure you have notes that include how and where you got it. (There is more about this later in this chapter in the discussion on how to do a complete reference.)

Internet Research

The Web opens access to scholarly (and not so scholarly) resources. For example, you may access directly, or through your university library, digital collections from around the world. You therefore can locate an enormous amount of material, but you need to proceed with caution and a critical eye. The Internet allows you to reach many credible resources (e.g., websites of health agencies and scientific organizations, and those useful peer-reviewed online journals). However, anyone can post anything on the Internet without review, screening, or adherence to standards, so be wary of the information you find because you can encounter misinformation and poor-quality research. Use your common sense about the authenticity and accuracy of the information before you incorporate it into your paper and do what you can to check the validity of a site and its authors. For example, many students often access Wikipedia—and we believe this is a great starting point. Much of its basic information is excellent, but some scientific and health information can be misleading or controversial because anyone can suggest content for the site (although it will go through an editorial screening panel). Wikipedia works to ensure validity of its information; however, many instructors prefer you obtain your resources from peer-reviewed professional sites.

When you search the Internet for resources pay careful attention to the domain names on Uniform Resource Locators (URLs); for example, URLs with extensions or suffixes such as.edu (educational institution), .gov (government), or .org (organization) usually lead you to reliable materials, but other domains may have biases and you should assess them critically.

When you visit and collect information from a credible website, be sure you make complete notes about the author(s), organization, address, date you visited the site, and the titles or headings of the sections or pages you used to obtain the information. Because it is so easy to block and print or save specific information from the Web, students often do not include the citation information that they will need later. Furthermore, many sites may be deleted or not accessible at a later date; check your Web addresses regularly.

Personal Communications

Sometimes you will obtain information from a specific individual; this is called a "personal communication" and includes interviews, letters, memos, telephone conversations, private Facebook pages, messages from non-archived discussion groups, email messages, or lectures from instructors. For a personal communication to mean something to your readers (audience), you (source) must provide enough information in your narrative to allow your reader to assess the value of this expert and the method you used to obtain the information. Always include the date of the communication and the person's initials and surname. Personal communications are mentioned in the text of your paper only (not in the reference list) unless the content is from a recoverable electronic communication, such as an archived discussion group. For example, suppose that you interviewed a clinical nurse specialist for a paper. The following illustrates two ways that you could identify this expert in the body of the paper:

A. J. Smith, clinical nurse specialist in the burn unit of Well Known Hospital, said an individual who experiences severe burns to a large portion of the body suffers profound physical and psychological shock (personal communication, December 5, 2018). She added that it usually is more important during the emergency period to deal first with the effects of shock (such as loss of fluids and emotional distress) than to start management of the burns themselves.

OR

Individuals who suffer severe burns to a large portion of the body suffer profound physical and psychological shock, and usually it is more important to deal first with the effects of shock than to start management of the burns (A. J. Smith, clinical nurse specialist, burn unit, Well Known Hospital, personal communication, December 5, 2018).

Personal communications also include information received by email. You asked an emergency health professional about care of burn patients and she emailed a reply. Make it clear in your message that you want to use the reply in your paper; some people do not like to have email responses or personal memos quoted. Some style manuals, and many instructors, suggest that you state this communication was received by email. So, for example, you might add a phrase into the citation in the body of your paper in this way:

... personal communication by email, December 5,......

Chapter 5 contains additional information about email messages.

CITING INFORMATION IN YOUR PAPER

So, in your assignment, you use a variety of resources. Now, you must acknowledge your indebtedness for the ideas and information you used. You do this both by citing your resource in the body of the message and by detailing it in a reference list or bibliography (at the end of a student paper).

More specifically, an *in-text citation* is used in the body of the paper to show where you used specific information from a particular resource; more information about that resource is given in the *reference list*. A *bibliography* is similar to the reference list but includes not only the resources used within the paper but also other materials consulted but not referred to directly in the paper. The reference list or bibliography allows readers to locate more detailed information on a point that interests them, to evaluate the credibility of the resource, or to verify your use of the information if it seems incorrect or controversial. Thus, you need to reveal not only who the expert is but how the reader can retrieve the materials.

Most of your references will likely be to recent books or professional journals, but some of them are hard to find without full details of when and where they were published. Some references (reports, theses, websites, papers presented at conferences) are almost impossible to find. Style guides or manuals provide rules about what specific information needs to be included in citations, references, and bibliographies and about how these informational details must be presented. (Style guides also provide many other rules, mentioned in other chapters of this book, such as when and how to use capital letters, how to punctuate, and which dictionary is recommended as a spelling guide.)

You use ideas or facts from your reference resources in two ways:

1. You acknowledge that the idea came from another resource but paraphrase it (i.e., put the idea in your own words, which must be substantially different from the words used in the original version).

2. You give the idea word for word as a direct quotation.

Either way, you must acknowledge your indebtedness to the resource. You need to make it clear that this was not your own, original idea but was thought of by someone else. You do this by indicating the resource in your paper near the point where it is mentioned; this practice is referred to as in-text citation. If you use information that was developed by someone else and you fail to acknowledge your dependence on this information, it is called "plagiarism," and it is a serious offence in the academic community.

PLAGIARISM

Plagiarism—use of another person's ideas or words without acknowledgement—can have grave consequences. In some instances, you may be given a mark of zero for the paper or suspended from the course. **You may even be expelled from a college or university for plagiarism.** Usually, the course calendar of your college or university contains a statement about plagiarism; you should read and remember this statement. You may also be provided with a handout stating your department's position on plagiarism.

Plagiarism is increasingly a matter of academic significance, and major articles have appeared in the news media about this kind of dishonesty. Technology has made it both easier to find instances of plagiarism and easier for you to commit plagiarism. Many colleges and universities now subscribe to computer programs, such as Turnitin or iThenticate; these programs can be used to scan student papers and identify exactly how much was copied or taken from other resources. Some instructors use such programs as teaching tools, usually in first-year courses, but have the program available in case they become concerned that a paper does not represent the student's own work. So please review your department's policies, be sure you understand what plagiarism is, and take great care in using references and citing them correctly. Being disciplined, or even expelled, for this kind of dishonesty may even affect your ability to become registered as a member of your profession.

The most serious kind of plagiarism, sometimes called complete plagiarism, is submission of a paper written by someone else for you. Complete plagiarism also includes using main ideas and large passages from one or more published works as the substance of your paper, even if you paraphrase the material and acknowledge your resources. Such practices generally represent attempts to cheat. Do not be tempted by writing services available online; this is cheating and it will result in serious damage to your education and your reputation. Some of these service providers offer a money back guarantee if you are caught; however this will not help you recover from the grave harm caused to your future.

Using a paper that you wrote for one course for another course is also unacceptable, even if you have modified it and updated the references and content; such a practice is called self-plagiarism. In some instances, you can build a new essay on information developed in an earlier paper, but you should obtain approval from your instructor first and, if requested to do so, provide a copy of the original paper. The new paper must represent more in-depth work, take a new approach, and be significantly different.

A more common instance of plagiarism results from sloppy note-taking during your reading or research or from failing to understand how to acknowledge the material you used. Take care when you copy passages from another's work and distinguish both ideas and phrases used in the original when you make your own statements. Because of the ease with which students can copy material from the Internet (email messages, files from others, pages downloaded from the Web) and put it into their own files, they sometimes lose track of what they copied and what they summarized themselves in notes. Keep good records and be sure you identify the original resource on all material you download. Instructors may find it hard to know whether such plagiarism was intentional or accidental. You may develop tricks for distinguishing messages copied and pasted from someone else during your research and brainstorming sessions—such as the use of a different typeface or italics.

Information regarded as common knowledge does not have to be supported. For example, if you have spent time in hospitals and have been fairly observant, you probably do not need to give a reference for the following idea: most registered nurses in Canada are women. But you know that your instructor would like you to support such observations.

In your reading, you have found an article titled "Men Nurses in Atlantic Canada," written by two professors from Memorial University, June Twomey and Robert Meadus. It was published on pages 78 through 88 in a 2016 issue of *The Journal of Men's Studies*. You see that although the article was published in 2016 it used statistics from 2014. This article clearly states that males in 2014 represented 6.6% of registered nurses in Canada and it also provided other interesting and relevant information about men in nursing. So you might decide to summarize some of the information as follows:

> About 93.4% of registered nurses working in Canada in 2014 were women, and numbers of men in nursing showed little increase.

However, you have to indicate where you found the information. You can just use the article by Twomey and Meadus—but you also can locate more recent statistics from a website maintained by the Canadian Nurses Association (CNA) that reports that in 2016, 7.8% of nurses were men. You also need to show where and how that article might be retrieved by your readers so that they can check your statistics or read more about it. If you are using the reference style most common in courses for health professionals, you could use the following format:

> In 2016, 92.2% of registered nurses working in Canada were women, and this number is slowly increasing (CNA, 2016; Twomey & Meadus, 2016).

Or you might write:

> Figures reported by the Canadian Nurses Association (2016) and by Twomey and Meadus (2016) show the percentage of registered male nurses in Canada slowly increased by 1.2% between 2014 and 2016.

In both examples, you are paraphrasing (rewording) material that was in the references. If you used some of the same wording from the article, however, you would need to put that information inside quotation marks, as in the following example:

> Twomey and Meadus (2016, p. 79), using 2014 data from Canadian Institute for Health Information, report "In Canada, nursing remains female concentrated with 6.6% of RNs being male." Data from a more recent 2016 Canadian Nurses Association report showed that the percentage of male nurses increased slowly between 2014 and 2016 (CNA, 2016).

Do you begin to see the differences?

If, from this brief explanation, you do not completely understand what plagiarism is and how to avoid it, then you need to do more research into that subject. Ask your instructor where you can find the statement on plagiarism used in your college or university and read it. Several articles available on the Internet also explain and give excellent—and sometimes lengthy—explanations of various types; see, for example, the websites on plagiarism for Florida State University (2017), Purdue University (2018), and Simon Fraser University (2017).

An important point to consider is that *you* and your readers must be able to distinguish your ideas from those you acquired in your reading and research. You also must organize your paper in an original manner and definitely not model its content on someone else's work. And you yourself must be able to distinguish between your own words and those of others and know within yourself when you are "borrowing," even if you paraphrase. "I did not know about that" is no excuse and may not be accepted by your instructors. If in doubt, acknowledge the resource.

In the three examples above, we have shown you one way to acknowledge information from others within the body of the paper (the in-text citation). You will also need a reference list at the end of the paper (or, in some courses, a footnote at the bottom of the page, depending on the style manual guidelines) that will provide information your readers need to find the original. But before you can decide how to identify the original resource in the text and how to set up the reference list, you need a bit more information. In the next section, we discuss the use of various reference styles.

REFERENCE STYLES

Style manuals are the vital aid to doing references. For example, they help you sort through ways to list materials you might use so that you, or your readers, can find them. Take a few minutes and look at the styles used in the readings for your courses.

Style manuals also deal with many minor points. For example, a small change related to the typing of a manuscript was decided between the third and fourth editions of the APA *Manual*. In the third edition, the APA *Manual* recommended that you use two spaces after punctuation that ends a sentence; in the fourth and fifth editions, it recommended that you should use a single space after punctuation at the end of a sentence. The two spaces after a period was a long-standing tradition taught in typing schools in the days of manual typewriters. Use of one space after the period broke with this tradition because computers now set type in a new way, but now many computer programs have reverted to putting two spaces after a period (even when this might be between initials or when it signals an abbreviation, such as Dr.). Usually, instructors will not notice this even if they are relatively strict about other points of style.

Another minor, but fundamental, change over time relates to use of the *hanging indent* for entries in reference lists. In the fourth edition of the APA *Manual*, the Association's editors changed from using the *hanging indent* to using paragraph style for items in the reference list, but they returned to the hanging indent in the fifth and sixth editions. Thus, you may see two styles of references, depending on which edition was used as a style guide for that article or textbook. The hanging indent style, which is now recommended by APA, looks like this:

> Zilm, G., & Perry, B. (2020). *An introduction to writing for health professionals: The SMART way* (4th ed.). Toronto: Elsevier Canada.

The paragraph style of indent, which was recommended in the fourth edition of the APA *Manual* and is recommended in some other style guides, looks like this:

> Zilm, G., & Perry, B. (2020). *An introduction to writing for health professionals: The SMART way* (4th ed.). Toronto: Elsevier Canada.

Do you see the differences?

Entries done in the hanging indent style are easier for readers to find and read than those in the paragraph style. We recommend that you learn to use the hanging indent style because you will need it throughout your career.

Style manuals deal with different types of reference listings (more than 150 different kinds). For example, there are *print books* (e.g., your textbook), but a book might be prepared by a single author, two authors, a group of authors, or issued under a "title" for the group of authors (e.g., the fictional "United Nations Committee on Health Regulations"). Alternatively, instead of the whole book having been written by an author or authors, it may be an edited book in which editors compile chapters written by experts in the discipline, perhaps including chapters or linking sections written by the editors themselves.

A book itself may have been issued only in a print or in a digital version (e.g., e-book, ePub, Kindle, PDF), or both. If you used the digital version, you will need to provide information on how to track it down on the Web, so you need its HTML, which usually appears at the end of a Web address, or its Digital Object Identifier (DOI). The HTML is the "home terminal" address for the web location. The DOI, issued by a United Nations international consultative committee, is a string of numbers, letters, and symbols that identify material and allow readers to access it easily.

If listing a book sounds difficult, the same challenges apply to articles, pamphlets, reports, websites, blogs, wikis, and other resources. You need to be able to access the required style manual that allows you to be consistent in your listings and is appropriate for your audience (in most of your early work, that means your instructor). Fortunately, your computer may be able to help you. Many universities and colleges subscribe to your required manual online and you can access it to guide you through the steps to format your listings. You just need to understand the principles for a complete and useful reference.

The most commonly used reference style for health professionals is that recommended in the Publication Manual of the American Psychological Association, or APA *Manual*, as noted in Chapter 1 (in the section about route). This manual was written by the staff of the American Psychological Association (APA, 2010) mainly for use by individuals who write articles for publication in health care and social science journals. The editors of these publications wanted their writers to be consistent in manuscripts. The sixth edition of this reference tool was published in 2010 by APA in Washington, DC. In 2016, the creators of the APA *Manual* developed a new electronic (cloud-based) resource called APA Style CENTRAL, now called Academic Writer (APA, 2019). Academic Writer is available by (expensive) subscription, but most colleges and universities subscribe to it for students and faculty. It includes digital learning guides, templates, and APA style tools that check for errors. One benefit of this electronic resource is that it allows for continuous updates, but the disadvantage is that it is difficult to keep abreast of new rules.

As well as guidance on grammar, punctuation, organization, and spelling, style guides outline rules you should follow to identify sources of information in your paper: the recommended reference style. These rules determine the way you mention the reference resources both in the body of the paper (in-text citations) and in the reference list or bibliography.

There are many, many ways of doing this, just as there are many styles of automobiles or shoes. The main purpose of an automobile is to provide transportation; the main purpose of shoes is to protect the feet; the main purpose of a reference is to enable a reader to find the original material. You need to know something about the various styles in use because you will see many different ones in your readings. For example, medical, chemistry, and biology journals tend to use reference styles markedly different from those in most health discipline journals.

Generally speaking, the following two main styles are used for references:

1. numerical style, in which a number—often a small, superscript number—is given within the text and the full information about each citation is listed at the end of the paper or occasionally at the bottom of the page, in numerical order; OR

2. author–year style, in which the names of the authors and the year the material was published are worked into the text, either in parentheses or within the sentence itself; the reference list at the end then contains the full resource information, with the items listed in alphabetical order according to the last name of the primary author.

The numerical style is used in *Canadian Nurse* and *American Journal of Nursing*, the professional nursing journals published in Canada and the United States by the professional associations, and it may be the style that you were taught in high school. This style is also used in many English courses. The author–year style, which is also called the Harvard method, is, with specific embellishments, the one recommended in the APA manuals; it is used in most journals for health professionals. Find out from your instructor which style you should use.

Drawing on the information about the Twomey and Meadus article mentioned above, an example of the numerical style is as follows:

About 93.4% of registered nurses working in Canada are women.[1]

Then, in the reference list at the end of the paper, or in a footnote at the bottom of the page, you would supply all details a reader would need to find the specific article containing the information; your citation would look something like this (depending on which style manual you used as a reference):

1. Twomey, JC, and Meadus, R. Men Nurses in Atlantic Canada. *The Journal of Men's Studies*, 2016, Vol.24, No.1, pp. 78–88.

If you were using the APA manuals, the information in the body of the paper would be given this way:

About 93.4% of registered nurses working in Canada are women (Twomey & Meadus, 2016).

The full information about the article in the reference list would be arranged alphabetically by author at the end of the paper and presented as follows:

Twomey, J.C., & Meadus, R. (2016). Men nurses in Atlantic Canada. *The Journal of Men's Studies, 24*(1), 78–88.

Please review carefully and compare the two examples of what might appear in the reference list. You will notice many minor differences between them, such as the use of periods in the initials, the use of the ampersand (&) versus spelling out *and*, the way capital letters are used in the title, the position of the publication year, the way the page numbers are given, the way the material is formatted within the paper, and so on. All these are "rules" of style that depend on which style manual is preferred by your audience, whether that audience is your instructor or the editors of a journal to which you want to submit your material.

Both the author–year style and the numerical style have strengths and weaknesses. The author–year method allows a knowledgeable reader to assess the importance of a reference without the tiresome chore of flipping to the end of the paper to see if the information comes from a well-known expert or from some esoteric source. As well, the reader can identify how recently the information was published or used; currency is particularly important in research papers. However, when many references are used, having the authors' names in the text can be bothersome for the reader. The numerical method is less distracting; the reader can concentrate on the message. The numerical method is particularly useful for short articles in which readers can quickly find the references.

How do you decide which style to use? Remember to think SMART. Have you been told by your instructor (audience) which style to use? Does the content (message) dictate the style? If you are writing for a newspaper or journal, what style does that publication (route) use? Which style do you (source) prefer? Notice which basic element was asked about first: audience. If your instructor has stated a preference, then you should use that style—or expect to lose marks! Check to see if the style is also used in other departments in your college or university, especially for courses in the humanities or the sciences; other departments may recommend other styles.

No matter what style is used, however, you will need to provide the full information that will enable a reader (or even you) to find the resource again. So, before you learn how to do your reference, you need to know what information constitutes a *complete citation*. Once you know that, you can apply the recommended style.

Exercise 3.1 Styles of References

Just to give you practice doing references and more feedback about specific points to watch, try using both the author–year style and the numerical style in the following simple exercise.

Imagine that you are writing a paper about health care students working together on a written assignment and you wish to include as a quotation the sentence "Interprofessional collaboration (IPC) improves communication between healthcare workers and healthcare delivery." You found this sentence in an article in the 2018 issue of *Nurse Education Today*; in volume 61, pages 36–42. The DOI is doi:10.1016/j.nedt.2017.11.005. The six-page article is titled "The role of personal resilience and personality traits of healthcare students on their attitudes towards interprofessional collaboration." It was written by a team of professors from occupational therapy, physical therapy, and nursing: Michal Avrech Bar; Michal Katz Leurer; Sigalit Warshawski; and Michal Itzhaki.

You want to incorporate this quote into your assignment somewhat along these lines:

> Although working together on written assignments can be time-consuming and frustrating, one article concluded that "interprofessional collaboration improves communication between healthcare workers and healthcare delivery."

Show how this sentence would be referenced in the text and how the full citation should appear in the list of references at the end of the paper. First try using the author–year style (following APA); then try using a numerical style.

Author–Year (APA) Style

> Text Paragraph
> Reference Listing

Numerical Style

> Text Paragraph
> Reference Listing

COMMENTS ON EXERCISE 3.1 STYLES OF REFERENCES

Your completed exercises should look something like these. You probably thought of a dozen questions as you began to work on this exercise, so you can see why you need to have access to a manual—and why managing references is a difficult task!

Author–Year (APA) Style

> Paragraph (in-text citation)
>
> Although working together on written assignments can be time-consuming and frustrating, one article concluded that "interprofessional collaboration improves communication between healthcare workers and healthcare delivery" (Avrech Bar, Katz Leurer, Warshawski, & Itzhaki, 2018, p. 236).
>
> Reference Listing (using hanging indent):
>
> Avrech Bar, M., Katz Leurer, M., Warshawski, S., & Itzhaki, M. (2018). The role of personal resilience and personality traits of healthcare students on their attitudes towards interprofessional collaboration. *Nurse Education Today, 61,* 36–42. doi:10.1016/j.nedt.2017.11.005.

Some of the points to note here:

- Note two of the authors have last names consisting of two words.
- Be sure the page number is given in the parentheses in the in-text citation because this is a direct quotation.
- Watch the position of the period at the end of the text; there are many specific rules, but in this case, a period does come after the reference.

- Use a capital only for the first word in the title of the article in the reference listing.
- Use capitals for all the main words in the name of the journal (a proper name).

Numerical Style Text

Paragraph (in-text citation)

Although working together on written assignments can be time-consuming and frustrating, one article on this subject concluded that "interprofessional collaboration improves communication between healthcare workers and healthcare delivery."[1]

Reference Listing (also uses a hanging indent style)

[1]. Avrech Bar, M., Katz Leurer, M., Warshawski, S., and Itzhaki, M. "The Role of Personal Resilience and Personality Traits of Healthcare Students on their Attitudes Towards Interprofessional Collaboration." *Nurse Education Today, 61,* 36–42 (2018). doi:10.1016/j.nedt.2017.11.005.

This is only **one** example of a style using numbers; you may have used, with the help of your reference tool, another that is acceptable. Some points to note about our numerical listing:

- The reference number used in the text could be in parentheses (1) or in brackets [1] rather than in superscript as shown. Note that the number may be a regular font or a superscript font in the listing; your computer program may decide this for you.
- The page number is not given in the text, only in the reference listing, and not all the page numbers of the article are included in this listing.
- The word *and* is spelled out in this style (& is used in APA style).
- The title of the article is inside quotation marks (some style manuals do not use quotation marks), and the first letters of all main words in the title are capitalized (again, this depends on the style manual).

A COMPLETE CITATION

Earlier in this chapter, we suggested that, as you gather information, you need to record accurate details about the source of every item you collect. Although you may not use every item you collect, you need to be able to give a full citation for all the material you use either in a *reference list* or in a *bibliography* (more about each of these later in this chapter). So, as you read and review each resource, make *complete* notes. Doing this is cumbersome initially, but once you get used to doing it, it makes your life easier and saves you time and frustration.

Complete citation information includes the following:

- full names of all authors or editors
- date of publication
- complete title of the book or other major resource (whether electronic or print)
- title of the chapter or section in a book (or other resource) if chapters are not all by the main author, editor, or group
- complete title of the journal (including number of the volume and, sometimes, the issue)
- other publishing information (such as place of publication and publisher)
- page numbers
- DOI or URL for some electronic materials

Each of these items will be discussed separately in more detail.

Name(s) of Author(s)

The most important information in identifying the source of the material you have used is the name or names of the author or authors. Your readers (particularly your instructors) will want to know these.

You have to note carefully all the names—and their order—given on materials you review. All professions have a few well-known names, and you will learn to recognize the important ones. A few style guides require you to use the full first names, but most (including APA) call for only the initials of the first names. But it is a good idea to include the full first names of all authors in your notes or on your copies because you may need them someday—and we recommend you get into this habit. You will probably be annoyed when you find an important article written by eight or more people, but you do need to record all the authors. Some style guides allow you to shorten the listing of authors above a certain number, usually more than six. You do this by using the phrase "et al.," an abbreviation for the Latin *et alii,* which means "and others."

The most appropriate place to find the names of the authors of the material you used in your research depends on the material itself. In a book, the best place to find the accurate names of the authors is usually the title page; avoid using the names as they appear on the cover because the names may appear there in a shortened form. The title page of the book is inside, often about three pages in, and contains the correct title and information about the edition number, which you may also need. Other information on the title page includes the name of the publisher and the city or cities where this publisher has its main offices—but more about these items later. The names of the authors of reports of limited circulation are often given only on the cover; there may or may not be a title page inside, so in those instances, you do take the names from the cover.

Sometimes the entire book is not written by the individuals named on the title page but contains sections or chapters written by others. Sometimes the individuals named on the title page are identified as editors or compilers; this means they determined the contents of the book and may have written some chapters but have asked others to contribute as well. In these cases, the names of the authors of the chapters usually will be given at the beginning of the chapter or at the beginning or end of the section. For example, a book called *Keeping Reflection Fresh: Top Educators Share Their Innovation in Health Professional Education* was compiled by editors Allan Peterkin and Pamela Brett-MacLean (published in 2016 by the Kent State University Press). Various chapters within the book are written by other experts. If, for example, you wanted to use material about using haiku as a reflective strategy from Chapter 10, you would have to acknowledge Beth Perry, Katherine Janzen, and Margaret Edwards as creators of this information; you would also have to acknowledge that this chapter (using its title) was in the book compiled by the two main editors (so this reference is going to get lengthy!). So, this means you need to note and record the authors (and the titles) of chapters or sections you use as well as the main authors or editors of the book. You can see why it is important to make notes about the details of the source.

Sometimes materials are produced or written by an organization or agency rather than an individual or group of individuals, and no name of a specific author or editor is given. The World Health Organization in Geneva, the American Psychological Association in Washington, the Canadian Nurses Association in Ottawa, and the Saskatchewan Lung Association in Regina are examples of organizations that issue publications. For such references, use the name of the organization as the author. Be sure you get the name of the organization right.

The names of the authors of a journal article are usually given at the beginning of the article; occasionally, especially in mass-circulation magazines such as *Time* or *Maclean's,* the name of the author is given at the end of the item. The author of an electronic resource, such as a blog or Facebook post, is usually easy to locate. Some webpages are written by individuals who write as members of a group. In these instances, you use the name of the group as the author in the reference. For television programs, films, and videos, you often use the name of the director in place of the author. This means taking care to read the credits at the beginning or end of the material.

Date of Publication

After the name(s) of the author(s), the next most important item to note for a complete citation is the date, usually the date the material was published (rather than the date the material was created or modified). The date of a publication gives you and your readers an excellent tip on how valuable the information might be. For example, if you were writing an article that mentioned the types of medications that might be ordered for a patient, an article that was 10 or more years old could be outdated. If, on the other hand, you found an article had historic information related to men in nursing, you might want to use it, but it would be important to find and add updated information. The article about males in nursing mentioned above may have been the best professional article available, but you would be able to add an additional reference with the latest data if a new census report became available.

For books, all you need to include in a complete citation is the year of publication (often called the copyright date). This information is sometimes given on the title page and sometimes only on the copyright page, which is usually the back of the title page. Sometimes a book goes through several editions, and several years may be listed on the copyright page; generally, you use only the most recent copyright date.

However, sometimes a book is republished and copyrighted again years after it was originally written, and you may need to make this clear in your citation (and in your paper). For example, Florence Nightingale's *Notes on Nursing* was written and originally published in 1859. It has been republished many times since; one facsimile edition was published in 1946 and is widely available. This might be the best possible reference for you to use in a paper on the history of nursing. But it could be confusing to some readers if you indicated 1946 for F. Nightingale (your readers might think there was another F. Nightingale), so you need to make the dates clear in your notes on the complete citation and, eventually, in the reference that you use in the paper.

For articles from periodicals (including journals, magazines, newspapers, regular statistical reports, and documents published several times annually), you need more than just the year; you may need the month and day. For many journals, this information is determined through the volume and, if necessary, the issue numbers. Because libraries used to bind issues of these journals, the volume number represented the number of issues that likely would be bound at one time, usually one year. Articles from professional journals often have the date, volume, and issue number on every page, so this would appear on any copies you might make or download. However, not all journals do this, and you may need to look elsewhere in the journal for this information. Usually, it is on the table of contents page, or on what is called the masthead, or, for some journals, only on the cover.

For information retrieved from online resources, you also need to include the date of "publication" or copyright, and sometimes finding this is tricky. Because the date (if there is one reported) can appear in a variety of locations, you may need to hunt for it. For example, the date on websites and some other online resources often appears at the top or near the end of the document; the publication date of a blog is usually with the author's name at the top. As a last resort, if a date cannot be found, use the no date option; just be careful because overuse of (n.d.) is frowned upon if it appears you are too lazy to look for it. Furthermore, online resources can be confusing because the "publication" date may change almost daily; however, a new date may mean there was a change in the format or design and not the substance.

You may find the dates for films, news clips, YouTube videos, TED talks, and such materials given in the credits at either the beginning or the end of a program. Dates for films are often given in Roman numerals (e.g., MCMLXXXVII, which is 1987); you may use either in your citation information, although Arabic numbers are recommended in APA style. You may also use the date on which you viewed a live (not recorded) television program, such as a news broadcast.

You also need to record dates for personal communications. This would be the date you interviewed your expert, the day you received the email, or the day the instructor mentioned the information in a class presentation. If the lecture material is not just general knowledge but specific information that must be attributed to the instructor as an expert, you will need to include the date in your paper. So get used to noting dates!

Titles

Titles are the next most important component in your complete citation or reference. Even listing a title can be fraught with problems. If you are referencing a book, then give its full title. Frequently, a book is referred to by only a portion of its title (e.g., *Notes on Nursing*), but its full title may have two or more parts (*Notes on Nursing: What It Is, and What It Is Not*). The title should be copied from the title page of the book rather than from the cover because the two sometimes differ; the one on the title page is the correct one. Note that you use the italic font for titles of books, as well as names of journals, films, ships, bacteria, and some other scientific terms. Some older style guides suggest you underline titles; that is because when typewriters were commonly used, they did not have an italic font. Use an underline to indicate titles when you are jotting handwritten notes.

The edition number may need to be included as a part of the title. A first edition usually is not specified on the title page (and so you need not give it); later editions are. Sometimes the title page shows that this is a revised edition, which is different from a second or third or fourth edition; in this case, you put the abbreviation in parentheses following the title but not in italics, this way: *Title of book* (Rev. ed.).

If the relevant material is from an article in a journal, then the title of the article is given as well as the title of the journal. Be sure you copy the full title of the journal correctly. Sometimes the name of a journal changes over the years. The original title of the official publication of the Canadian Nurses Association was *The Canadian Nurse.* In the 1960s, when the journal became a bilingual publication, its name was *The Canadian Nurse / L'infirmière canadienne.* In 1999, when the journal once again began to be published in separate English and French editions, the name of the English version was changed again, this time to *Canadian Nurse* (without *The*).

In most student papers, these minor distinctions would not matter; you could simply use *Canadian Nurse,* and your readers—including your instructor—would certainly be able to locate the journal. However, some routes (professional journals) and some audiences (including some instructors) want to see the distinctions, so you would be wise to note carefully the exact name when you are making notes about the material you wish to use.

Various electronic resources, such as Facebook pages, streaming videos including YouTube or Vimeo, or Twitter pages, also usually have titles that need to be part of your complete citation. You include the title in the same location in the reference as you do in books and articles, but you indicate the type of resource in square brackets after the title. For example, if the title of a YouTube video was *How to learn to spell complicated drug names* you would write *How to learn to spell complicated drug names* [Video file] as the title.

Other Information for Retrieval

In addition to those three most important items—names of authors, dates of publication, and accurate titles—a few other bits of information are needed for a complete citation so that a reader can find and retrieve the original. These other items concern the place of publication or production, name of the publisher or sponsor, page numbers, and in some cases the DOI or URL.

For books, information for a complete citation includes the name of the company that published the material and the city where the publishing company has its headquarters. Usually, this information is contained on the title page of the book. You may find that the company's name is followed by a long list of cities; you do not need to list all these, only the one where the book was produced (usually the first one in the list), and you can find or verify that information on the copyright page. For example, some publishers have their major headquarters in the United States or the Netherlands, but their Canadian books are published through the Canadian head office.

If the city is well known, you are not required to give the province or state, unless there is likely to be some confusion. For example, a few Canadian publishers are in London, Ontario; you need to distinguish this city from London, England. Almost all style guides now recommend that writers use the standard abbreviations recommended by the post office for province, state, or country, which is available on the inside back cover of this text and is also easily available online. Thus, for London, Ontario, you would use London, ON; you do not need to put London, UK (for United Kingdom), because readers should assume that it is the major world city. You would put Oxford, UK, however, to distinguish it from Oxford, NY (for New York). You also need to think SMART with the cities. If you are writing in Canada for a Canadian audience, then you probably could put Saskatoon rather than Saskatoon, SK; if you are writing for an American journal, however, you would be wise to designate the province.

You can use a shortened version of the publisher's name if the publisher is a major one. Thus, you could just put "Merriam" rather than "G. & C. Merriam Company." You will soon catch on to your commonly used textbook publishers. Take a look at references and bibliographies in a couple of your texts to see variations in style and kinds of information most commonly used. If the publisher is a small house or a small agency, unknown to the general public, you may also need to give a full address, although this is rare in student papers.

You also need to identify the city and the name of the publisher for reports and other published documents. Often these are published by associations, such as the American Physical Therapy Association. Some of the documents you will use for your papers may be published by government agencies or departments, and styles for the citation of government documents can be tricky. For printed materials available only in limited forms, such as pamphlets or reports by some small local agencies, there are special rules, such as inclusion of a street address for a local agency. Again, copy as much information as you can about the sponsoring organization into your notes so that you will have it when you complete your paper. Include as much information as possible from the cover or from the title page and copyright page; when you come to use the material in your paper, you can then check on how to cite the information based on the style guide that you will use.

If you are taking information from the Internet, be sure you make full, complete notes on the Web address; sometimes this is included on the printout or downloaded document, but sometimes it is not. You also should make complete notes on—or print out or download—the homepage of the resource, which will give you information that may be necessary for your reference. For example, if you print out a section on "professional images" from a work that has the (fictional) address <http://www.amu.bc.ca/>, you might not be aware that the section was from a document called "Attributes of a Professional" and that the "author" was the Engineering Department of the Alma Mater University in Surrey, British Columbia; however, all that information should be in your complete citation.

For films, television programs, and videos, all you usually need is the city and the name of the production company (such as MGM of Hollywood, California, or WarnerMedia in New York). CDs and DVDs usually provide this information on the disc itself. Many electronic resources such as blog posts, podcasts, or web pages will not have a city of publication or a publisher, but you will need to provide the URL or the DOI from these types of materials. You may ask, How do I know when to use a DOI and when the URL is the correct choice to create a complete citation? It is complicated, but there are some basic rules to guide you. If possible, include a DOI as it is unique to each item of content and is considered a persistent link, which means it should lead people to the resource you used. When no DOI is available, include the URL. Remember your goal is to provide a simple and direct means for your audience to locate your references.

For personal communications, it usually is not necessary to give the name of the city. If you are using information obtained from a printed version of a speech, however, you would include this in the reference list and identify the organization for which the speech was prepared and the city in which the speech was presented.

The last bit of relevant information that you should be sure you have for a complete citation is page numbers. This is especially important if you intend to quote from the material. Page numbers for books and articles are usually easy to find, even if you photocopy or download them for later use. Just be sure, however, that the page number actually appears on the photocopy or download. For example, the opening page of a chapter in some books does not have a page number; if you copied only that page so that you would have the exact wording for a quotation, you would not find it when you came to complete your paper. Photocopies or downloads from large pages, such as newspaper pages, often do not show the page number; be sure to note the page number on your copy. A few books, such as small books of poetry or catalogues, do not have page numbers; in these cases, you must do a rough count of the pages (often referred to as "leaves" and abbreviated in the citation as l.) and note the number on the copy.

So, you see, making the notes for a complete citation when you are doing your research involves a lot of details. Get into good habits early!

BIBLIOGRAPHIES VERSUS REFERENCE LISTS

Do you know the difference between a reference list and a bibliography? A *reference list* (frequently entitled "References" in your subheading) contains all documents you used in the paper (cited in-text) and they are listed in alphabetical order. A *bibliography* contains all the documents that you reviewed to help you understand the content, even if you have not actually cited them in the paper; they are also listed alphabetically. Both lists are based on the complete notes you made during your reading and research.

Thus, you may need two lists at the end of your paper. A bibliography is usually much longer and more complete than a reference list and may include general texts or style guides. If you did not use ideas or information from any books or journals in the body of the paper (highly unlikely for student papers), you would not even need a reference list. You might, however, want to acknowledge the various resources that you reviewed, and so you would have a bibliography.

Graduate students preparing theses or dissertations (route) and authors of books may need both a reference list and a bibliography. Because journals (a different route) usually want to keep the lists attached to the articles as short as possible, editors of most journals want only a reference list. APA style manuals do not even have detailed information about bibliographies because the manuals were developed for editors and authors of journals. So, in APA style, students could combine the two lists into one (and call it References). Check with your instructors (audience) as well because some like only a reference list that shows the information on the in-text citations and some do not like to see combined lists. Other style guides, especially those using the numerical style, call for different layouts for the two lists.

There is also another kind of bibliography—an *annotated bibliography*. This list can be set up using the basic style that your instructor (audience) wants and that you would use for the reference list at the end of your paper.

However, after each entry, you provide a brief note (annotation) about the material that gives additional information for the reader; you may even include some material that did not seem relevant for the body of the paper. You also may add your own comments about the merits or limitations of the material. Annotated bibliographies are frequently assigned in more senior courses and are often used as the basis for a literature review. A literature review is done by senior researchers and often contains not only an exhaustive bibliographical list of resources relevant to the topic but also a narrative report in which the writer compares and contrasts the information in various resources and is able to come up with new conclusions. Even some of your early assignments in your courses may be elementary types of such a literature search.

You may also need some feedback about how you use references so that you can learn to do them better. One excellent way of obtaining such feedback is to exchange a list of references with another student in one of your health profession courses and then spend a few minutes critiquing them for each other.

We strongly recommend that, as you do your reading and research, you begin to create your own bibliographical database for current and future assignments. You can do this manually, or you can access one of several citation or reference management tools available online that will guide you to make complete citations, help you organize your references, and create reference lists and bibliographies in a variety of styles. Most of these tools are searchable in several ways, including by keywords. Many of these tools are free, or at least free within certain limits such as amount of storage or included features. You can use your collection of references to share with others or you can access it to create specific reference lists or bibliographies for your assignments. The programs will automatically generate reference lists using one of the common reference styles. If you begin using one of these tools early in your program, it will save you time and aggravation searching for reference details later. Zotero, Mendeley, RefWorks, and EndNote are examples of such electronic reference management tools. Most tools create output styles that will match the style you are required to use in your assignments (e.g., APA, MLA, Harvard). Choose the reference management tool that works for you. If you need a more advanced version (one that is not free), check with your college or university library to see if you can obtain student access because some campuses purchase a license for common reference management tools. Discuss the different ones with other students and instructors who use them. And a final word of warning: Sometimes, automatically generated references may be inaccurate, so you do need to have an understanding of the principles (see Box 3.1).

BOX 3.1   General Principles for APA Style Reference Lists

- Begin "References" on a new page at the end of the paper; this subtitle is centred.
- Use only references listed in your paper (in-text citations), unless otherwise requested to do so by your instructor. (And then, technically, this would be headed "References and Bibliography.")
- Double-space throughout, but do not put an additional space between entries.
- Use the "hanging indent"; first line of an entry is at the left margin and all following lines of the entry are indented one-half inch (five spaces).
- Arrange the list alphabetically by the last names of the author(s) or editor(s) in the order these are shown on title page or near the top of the material; if more than one reference has the same first author, a single-author entry precedes multi-author entries.
- Use surnames of authors or editors followed by initials (not full first name). When there are two or more surnames, separate the name (and its initials) by commas and use an ampersand (&) before the last author's name. Include a space between authors' initials if more than one initial (i.e., Brown, J. A.). This segment of the listing is closed by a final period.
- For two or more works by the same author, arrange entries by earliest year first; if there are two or more works by the same author or editor (or the *exact same* group of authors listed in the same order) published the same year, then add a lowercase a or b or c following the year (e.g., 2019a) and list them in alphabetical order by the first major word in the title (omitting "a" or "an" or "the"). This happens more often than you might expect!
- Place, within parentheses and by a period to indicate the closing of this segment, the year the material you used was published following the names of the author(s) or editor(s); for articles in magazines and newspapers, use the full date (year, followed by month and number of the day) in the reference list: (e.g., 2019a, July 7).
- If there is no year, use n.d. (meaning "no date") in parentheses.

Continued

BOX 3.1   General Principles for APA Style Reference Lists—Cont'd

- If a work has no author or editor, move the title to the author position and list alphabetically by the first major word of the title (again omitting "a" or "an" or "the").
- Put titles (and, if necessary, subtitles as listed on the title page) of the main work in italics, but do not italicize article or chapter titles.
- Capitalize only the first word of the title and subtitle (and all proper nouns) and the first word of the subtitle. Capitalize names of periodicals as you would capitalize them normally as these are considered "proper names."
- Put abbreviations for "page" and "pages" ("p." and "pp.") for journal and newspaper articles or for chapters (sections) in edited books. It is not necessary to put page numbers for material from websites.
- For professional journals and other such serials, page numbers—without use of "p." and "pp."—are placed following the volume number (and, if necessary, the issue number).
- If there is a Digital Object Identifier (DOI), which provides a persistent link to its location on the Internet, list it following the main entry.
- If the material was obtained on the Internet and does not have a DOI, include the full HTML listing after the main entry. (Reference to the database is no longer necessary with a DOI.)
- If you are doing an annotated bibliography, add your brief note or the abstract in block format after the citation but starting on a new line and indented a further two spaces.

Refer to Box 3.2 below and to the References at the end of each chapter for this textbook, and you will find examples illustrating these principles.

COMMON ERRORS IN REFERENCES

Students often make three specific errors when they are doing references in their papers: failure to cite the relevant chapter, inappropriate use of secondary resources, and failure to introduce quoted material into the paper in a way that does not break the flow of the narrative.

Failure to Cite the Relevant Chapter

A number of students make the mistake of referring to a book when they should be referring to a relevant chapter. If the whole book was written by a single author or a group of authors, then one reference will do. However, today many textbooks are compiled by one or more editors and contain chapters written by different authors.

The following is an example of an **incorrect** reference (using a fictional citation):

> Great writers have a creative style and are not afraid to be original (Mino, 2019, p. 47).

Although your instructor can refer to this resource and check your findings or get further information (basic purposes of a citation), this is not the way that the author–year method is done.

In the example given, George Mino is the editor of a text that includes chapters written by him and some chapters by other expert authors. The information in this sentence actually comes from Chapter 3, titled "Creative Strategies for Becoming a Great Writer," by Kerry Andle alone, and, as author, he is the only one who should be mentioned in this citation. Thus, the correct way to format this in-text citation is the following:

> Great writers have a creative style and are not afraid to be unique (Andle, 2019, p. 47).

In the reference list, the full citation, using APA style, would read:

> Andle, K. (2019). Creative strategies for becoming a great writer. In G. Mino (Ed.), *Writing for rookies* (pp. 35–50). Small City, NB: Inventive Press.

You may need to give a separate citation for the whole Mino book in the bibliography (or in a combined references and bibliography listing). The bibliographical mention of the book would indicate that you at least browsed through it and may have read several other chapters that were not specifically cited. You may need to list several chapters from the book in the reference list. Doing so may seem to make your reference list longer than necessary, but it represents the correct way to list materials from an edited text. This method is clear for your readers, and it gives the credit to the real authors of the information.

Citing Secondary Resources

Use of secondary resources can create problems in student papers. A secondary resource means that you are referring to a text (and its author) cited in another text, but you have not gone back to check the original. *Occasionally* this is permissible, but students should not do it routinely, and not without good reason. (The fact that you cannot obtain the original is sometimes an acceptable reason, but now many outdated books are easily available online so this reason has become less acceptable.)

A main reason you should not use secondary resources is that the primary resource (i.e., the author you read) might not have used the original material correctly or might have used it out of context. When you also use it without seeing the original, the error often gets compounded. So either go to the original or cite the material correctly as a secondary resource.

Another alternative is to word the information so that you need not cite the primary resource; you have to do this carefully and accurately, of course. You need to note the original author and may need to note when the original work was published.

The following example illustrates this point. In England in 1859, Florence Nightingale wrote: "Bad sanitary, bad architectural, and bad administrative arrangements often make it impossible to nurse." This passage was published the same year in London in a little book called *Notes on Nursing*. This book was republished in the United States in 1860. You read in a recent textbook (we made this one up), written by Ann Author, that quotes this passage from Florence Nightingale. In your paper, you might want to use this quotation to illustrate that some common health care problems have been around for many years, but you cannot find an online copy of the rare Florence Nightingale book to check the original quote. So you might use only the secondary resource, showing the in-text citation in your paper this way:

> Health care professionals have long recognized that poor conditions in the workplace can affect the kind of care given. Florence Nightingale, in 1859, recognized these problems, writing that "bad sanitary, bad architectural, and bad administrative arrangements often make it impossible to nurse" (as cited in Author, 2021, p. 87).

You would then list only the secondary resource in the reference list at the end of your paper, thus:

> Author, A. (2021). *Quoting Florence: An old book for modern times*. Wild Oaks, CA: Reliable Press.

"Sticking In" Quotations

Be careful about "sticking in" a quotation, even if you believe that it illustrates your point well. Sometimes you can do it and the reader can immediately understand the logic behind the quotation. Most times, however, you improve the flow of your writing if you "lead in" to the quotation. Here is a completely fictional example of a poor way to use a quotation:

> Nurses need to be able to communicate well. "All nurses need a master's degree in English grammar" (Zilm, 1923, p. 34). Poor communications can confuse patients.

This quotation may mislead the reader. Are you advocating that nurses need to have degrees in English but using words from Zilm to back up your idea? The following revision helps to clear up that question and it improves the flow:

> Nurses need to be able to communicate well. Writing fanatic Gwennyth Zilm (1923) even suggested that "All nurses need a master's degree in English grammar" (p. 34). Poor communications can confuse patients.

You may have noticed in some books that each chapter starts with a quotation. This literary device dates back hundreds of years and is a good, creative way to get readers thinking. However, that is a special literary method and usually does not have a place within a paragraph, in which each sentence must flow from one to the other in a way that the reader can follow easily. So when you use a quotation within a paragraph, make it clear how it ties in with the previous sentence.

BOX 3.2 Working Bibliography (using the resources mentioned in this chapter—real and fictitious)

Annotated Working Bib for my Nursing 101 course

(*Note to self: These references are based on APA style but are not formatted correctly; check the style before pasting one of these resources into a paper.*)

Andle, K. (2019). Creative strategies for becoming a great writer. In G. Mino (Ed.), *Writing for rookies* (pp. 35–50). Small City, NB: Inventive Press.

> A book of helpful hints for new writers. Could be helpful in cases of writer's block when looking for a good way to start or end a paper or if I have a professor who seems to appreciate creativity in assignments.

Author, A. (2021). *Quoting Florence: An old book for modern times.* Wild Oaks, CA: Reliable Press.

> Fictional book with quotes from Florence Nightingale. Could be useful in nursing assignments. Context for quotes provided.

Avrech Bar, M., Katz Leurer, M., Warshawski, S., & Itzhaki, M. (2018). The role of personal resilience and personality traits of healthcare students on their attitudes towards interprofessional collaboration. *Nurse Education Today, 61,* 36-42, doi:10.1016/j.nedt.2017.11.005

> A research-based paper from a peer-reviewed journal that provides a good foundation for understanding the value of interprofessional collaboration in quality healthcare. [Note that some of the author surnames are two words.]

Canadian Nurses Association. (2016). *Registered nurses profile (including nurse practitioners), Canada.* Retrieved from https://cna-aiic.ca/en/on-the-issues/better-value/health-human-resources/nursing-statistics/canada

> Includes statistics related to registered nurse and nurse practitioner supply and workforce, demographic profile, and employment location and positions. All statistics relate to Canadian nurses and are from 2016. Provides only nursing stats, but similar sites are available for other health professionals.

Clarivate Analytics (2017). Endnote. Retrieved from http://endnote.com/

> Homepage includes details about this reference management software that helps with formatting reference lists and bibliographies. Gives details about how to sign up for a free trial.

BOX 3.2   Working Bibliography (using the resources mentioned in this chapter—real and fictitious)—Cont'd

Nightingale, Florence. (1946/1859). *Notes on nursing: What it is and what it is not.* Philadelphia: Lippincott. (Facsimile edition; original published in 1859) (Available from http://en.wikisource.org/wiki/Notes_on_Nursing:_What_It_Is,_and_What_It_Is_Not)

    An invaluable classic resource. Although Nightingale was a nurse, her notions have application for all types of health professionals. Though it was written in 1859 the ideas are relevant.

Perry, B., Edwards, M., & Janzen, K. (2016). Haiku it! – Reflection in 17 syllables. In A. Peterkin & P. Brett-MacLean (Eds.), *Keeping reflection fresh: Top educators share their innovations in health professional education* (pp. 23–25). Kent, OH: Kent State University Press.

    A chapter from an edited book with contributions by many authors, most of them university professors. Gives wonderful examples about writing and using haiku. As well, the ideas in the rest of the book are useful for assignments about teaching health professionals.

RefWorks (2019). RefWorks. Retrieved from https://www.refworks.com/refworks2/default.aspx?r=authentication::init

    Useful homepage for the reference management tool RefWorks. Includes a quick start guide and video tutorials. I can access other pages with information on RefWorks. For example, Proquest RefWorks has a series of YouTube videos for people new to RefWorks.

    Proquest RefWorks (n.d.). RefWorks video tutorials. Retrieved from https://www.youtube.com/user/ProQuestRefWorks

Twomey, J., & Meadus, R. (2016). Men nurses in Atlantic Canada. *The Journal of Men's Studies, 24*(1),78–88. doi:10.1177/1060826515624414

    A research report written by professors from Memorial University. Uses 2014 statistics. Valuable for assignments related to gender issues in health care (especially nursing).

Zilm, G., & Perry, B. (2020). *An introduction to writing for health professionals: The SMART way* (4th ed.). Toronto: Elsevier Canada.

    Excellent resource to guide writing of assignments. A resource to use throughout my program. Includes an abundance of helpful and practical information.

POINTS TO REMEMBER

❑ You need to become skilled in locating credible, reliable, and well-chosen resources to use in assignments.

❑ You need to learn to read critically for style as well as content.

❑ You need to know how to use a style manual to assist you with citations, references, and bibliographies. Good style is like good care for patients—you do not particularly notice it when it is good, but you notice it when it is bad!

❑ You need to know the background and general principles for use of APA style; this chapter, however, is not intended as a substitute for current APA manuals (whether hardcopy or online).

❑ You need to be aware that preparing written assignments with appropriate in-text citations and accurate reference lists can be a tricky business!

REFERENCES

American Psychological Association. (2010). *Publication manual of the American Psychological Association* (6th ed.). Washington, DC: Author.

American Psychological Association. (2019). *Academic Writer* [website]. Retrieved from http://digitallearning.apa.org/academic-writer

Avrech Bar, M., Katz Leurer, M., Warshawski, S., & Itzhaki, M. (2018). The role of personal resilience and personality traits of healthcare students on their attitudes towards interprofessional collaboration. *Nurse Education Today*, *61*, 36–42. https://doi.org/10.1016/j.nedt.2017.11.005

Canadian Nurses Association. (2016). Registered nurses profile (including nurse practitioners), Canada. Retrieved from https://www.cna-aiic.ca/en/nursing-practice/the-practice-of-nursing/health-human-resources/nursing-statistics

Clarivate, Analytics. (2017). *Endnote*. Retrieved from http://endnote.com

Florida State University. (2017). *Plagiarism*. Retrieved from http://guides.lib.fsu.edu/plagiarism

iThenticate. (2018). *Prevent plagiarism in published works*. Retrieved from http://www.ithenticate.com/

Mendeley. (2019). *Mendeley*. Retrieved from https://www.mendeley.com/?interaction_required=true

Nightingale, F. (1946). *Notes on nursing: What it is and what it is not*. Philadelphia: Lippincott. (Original published in 1859).

Perry, B., Edwards, M., & Janzen, K. (2016). Haiku it! – Reflection in 17 syllables. In A. Peterkin & P. Brett-MacLean (Eds.), *Keeping reflection fresh: Top educators share their innovations in health professional education* (pp. 23–25). Kent, OH: Kent State University Press.

Proquest RefWorks. (n.d.). RefWorks video tutorials [Videos]. Retrieved from https://www.youtube.com/user/ProQuestRefWorks

Purdue University. (2018). *Avoiding plagiarism*. Retrieved from https://owl.purdue.edu/owl/teacher_and_tutor_resources/preventing_plagiarism/avoiding_plagiarism/index.html

RefWorks. (2019). *RefWorks*. Retrieved from https://refworks.proquest.com/.

Simon Fraser University. (2017). *Avoiding plagiarism*. Retrieved from https://www.lib.sfu.ca/help/academic-integrity/plagiarism

Turnitin. (n.d.). *Education with integrity*. Retrieved from https://www.turnitin.com

Twomey, J. C., & Meadus, R. (2016). Men nurses in Atlantic Canada: Career choice, barriers, and satisfaction. *The Journal of Men's Studies, 24*(1), 78–88. https://journals.sagepub.com/doi/10.1177/1060826515624414

Zilm, G., & Perry, B. (2020). *An introduction to writing for health professionals: The SMART way* (4th ed.). Toronto: Elsevier Canada.

Common errors are simple, everyday mistakes that you often find in the writings of nonprofessional writers—and even in the writings of some professional writers. You may hear some of these mistakes daily on your radio and television or read them in the popular press or magazines. You may even hear them in conversation with your instructors or in lectures. Think for a minute, however, about the SMART elements: usage is affected by route. The errors discussed in this chapter are elementary ones that you should not make in formal college- or university-level assignments.

Frequently, these common errors represent things that you can say (use appropriately, even in formal *oral* communications) but that are not appropriate in formal written communications. You may have heard the maxim "Write the way you talk"; that piece of good advice tells you to avoid seeming too pretentious. However, unless you have learned to use correct grammar and to speak fluent and correct English, you probably need to make some effort to write slightly more formally in your assignments than you normally speak. For example, many teenagers today routinely say "Me and George are going to the store"; however, this would identify even an undergraduate student as one who is uneducated and careless. You should also avoid contractions (e.g., *I'm, we've, can't, won't, shouldn't, it's*) in college or university work unless you are quoting from another source or reproducing dialogue. So, when you are editing your assignments, you need to look for these everyday errors.

In Chapter 2, we described the steps of the writing PROCESS, concentrating on how to **P**lan, **R**esearch, and **O**rganize your information, and on how to begin to **C**reate a first draft. We also mentioned the steps of **E**diting, **S**hining up your prose, and **S**ubmitting your paper. In this chapter, we discuss common errors you will find, especially during those editing and polishing steps—the ones you do after you have developed and drafted the content of your paper to your satisfaction.

Although this chapter deals with some errors in grammar, our text is not intended to be a basic grammar book. If you have been accepted into a college or university program, you are expected to have good language, grammar, and writing skills. As mentioned in Chapter 1, you should have, as reference tools, access to a good dictionary and one or two good basic grammar resources (an online editing tool or grammar checker) to help you as you edit, revise, and polish. Just how basic or how advanced your reference tools should be will depend on your present skills as a writer; choose the kind of aid you need now, but be prepared to look for more advanced support as you gain better writing skills through practice, reading, and feedback from your instructors.

You need to correct the following common errors before you type up the final version. Allow yourself about an hour to go through the final draft, looking for these 12 common errors:

- long, complex sentences
- passive (rather than active) voice
- weak pronouns and verbs to begin sentences
- long, complicated, or inappropriate words (jargon)
- lack of agreement of terms
- lack of parallel structure
- misused words
- biased language
- unnecessary words
- inconsistencies in punctuation, spelling, and capitalization
- misuse of i.e. and e.g.
- poor paragraphing

COMMON ERROR: LONG, COMPLEX SENTENCES

Communication today has become a science, and a great deal of research has been done into what classic communication researcher Rudolf Flesch (1911–86) called "readability" (Flesch, 1960). Such research shows that people with high school and university educations are most comfortable reading sentences that average about 20 to 25 words. When a sentence contains 40 or more words, even people with doctoral degrees tend to get confused and disoriented, although if they are familiar with the subject matter, they can often follow the ideas. Clear words, logical flow, and good punctuation also help a reader to get through the maze. However, long sentences make readers tired and irritable. Do you want an irritable instructor marking your paper?

Reading your paper aloud often helps you to spot long sentences, although you can also find them simply by looking at the final draft. Usually, you can divide long sentences into two (or more) shorter sentences that convey your thoughts more clearly. You do not want to make all your sentences short; doing so will make your paper sound like a primary school assignment. Just take care that a sentence is not too long and that there are not many long sentences. Look critically at some of the articles you are required to read. When you need to reread passages because you seem to lose the meaning, you will usually find that a long sentence is the culprit.

Exercise 4.1 Long, Complex Sentences

Try reading the following long sentence, which appeared in a draft report written for the American Hospital Association.

> In addition to their primary mission of providing health care and related education to the sick and injured, hospitals have a responsibility to work with others in the community to assess the health status of the community, identify target health areas and population groups for hospital-based and cooperative health promotion programs, develop programs to help upgrade the health in those target areas, and ensure that persons who are apparently healthy have access to information about how to stay well and prevent disease, provide appropriate health education programs that aid those persons who choose to alter their personal health behavior or develop a more healthful lifestyle, and establish the hospital within the community as an institution which is concerned about good health as well as one concerned with treating illness.

Try rewriting the message to make it clearer. Then, refer to the following comments for suggestions.

COMMENTS ON EXERCISE 4.1 LONG, COMPLEX SENTENCES

That sentence had 129 words in it. You could rewrite its message in several ways. The 119 words in the following version are divided into five sentences (two of which use semicolons, which help to turn the sentences into seven distinct thoughts); thus, this version is much easier to understand.

> In addition to a primary mission of providing care and related education to the sick and injured, hospitals have four goals. First, hospitals need to work with local individuals to assess the community's health status. Second, hospitals must help identify target health areas and population groups for hospital-based and cooperative health-promotion programs; they then develop programs to help upgrade health in those target areas. Third, hospitals also must ensure that apparently healthy persons have access to information about how to stay well and prevent disease; hospitals must provide appropriate health-education programs that aid

people to alter their health behaviors and develop healthful lifestyles. Fourth, hospitals must be community institutions just as concerned with good health as with treating illness.

The following passage uses a different format to break up the message and make it easier for the reader to follow. It contains 125 words in the sentence, but the message is broken into distinct parts and is therefore easier to read.

In addition to the primary mission of providing health care and related education to the sick and injured, hospitals have six other goals:
- to work with others in the community to assess the health status of the community;
- to identify target health areas and population groups for hospital-based and cooperative health-promotion programs;
- to develop programs to help upgrade health in those target areas;
- to ensure that persons who are apparently healthy have access to information about how to stay well and prevent disease;
- to provide appropriate health-education programs that aid those persons who choose to alter their personal health behavior or develop a more healthful lifestyle; and
- to be an institution within the community that is as concerned with good health as with treating illness.

However, this last example uses "point form," which some instructors frown upon--especially if used excessively.

COMMON ERROR: PASSIVE RATHER THAN ACTIVE VOICE

Use of active voice in writing gives strength and vitality to a sentence; passive voice slows things down. Passive voice is when the doer of the action in the sentence is not the subject of the main verb. Communication research shows that passive voice is more confusing and tiring for readers. Consider the following examples:

- A splendid coach was pulled by six black horses.
- The bed was pushed across the room.
- My first visit to Well Known Hospital will always be remembered.

The first example is not a major problem for readers. The sentence is short and clear. Occasional use of such passive sentences is fine because they may give variety to your essay. The second example illustrates how passive voice creates problems that may be more serious. Ask yourself: "Pushed across the room by whom? Does the reader need to know this information?" In many instances, the reader does need to know such information; even if the reader does not need to know it, he or she might wonder who did the pushing and thereby become distracted from your real message. The last example illustrates the kind of problem that occurs when writers misuse passive voice; the meaning of the sentence is not clear. Ask yourself, "Remembered by whom?" The writer of that sentence probably meant "I will always remember my first visit to Well Known Hospital," although another meaning is certainly possible.

Some writers, including many researchers, tend to use (and misuse) passive voice in attempts to keep themselves in the background. In recent years, researchers use first-person pronouns (*I* or *we*) when necessary or to avoid passive voice. If they do not, they may get into difficulty with the meanings of sentences. In professional documents, technical reports, or routes other than an essay or formal paper, you may be advised to "keep yourself out of the writing." However, you can still avoid passive voice and keep yourself in the background. Look at the following two sentences:

- Some statistics were found to be extraneous to the report but were put into Appendix A. (Passive—found by whom? put by whom?)
- Some statistics did not apply to this report but are in Appendix A. (Active)

The solution is to use active voice whenever you can. Watch for passive voice when you are checking your final drafts and change it when necessary.

Note that passive voice and past tense are different. A sentence in the active voice can be in the past tense. If you do not understand the difference, then refer to this point in a good basic grammar resource.

Try the following exercise.

Exercise 4.2 Passive Rather Than Active Voice

In this exercise, sentences are in the passive voice; rewrite each one in the active voice:

1. A memo to unit managers, advising them of the workshop, was sent by the vice-president of patient care.

2. A copy of each prescription must be sent back to the unit with the drug from Pharmacy.

An Introduction to Writing for Health Professionals: the SMART way

3. The agenda for the meeting should be prepared by the representative from Rehabilitation Therapy.

4. The purchasing department door was left unlocked by someone; this made it possible for the computer records to be picked up by mistake when the delivery person made his rounds.

5. Fire regulations must be explained to each new employee during orientation week.

6. As he entered the hospital, the chairman of the board was hit on the head by a flowerpot falling from the window ledge above the door.

COMMENTS ON EXERCISE 4.2 PASSIVE RATHER THAN ACTIVE VOICE

Most of these sentences could be rewritten in a number of ways, but the following show some of the easiest ways to repair each one. Think about each rewritten version. Is the active voice better in all revisions?

1. The vice-president of patient care sent a memo to unit managers, advising them of the workshop.

   OR

   The unit managers received a memo, advising them of the workshop, from the vice-president of patient care.

In the original sentence, the main verb is part of "to send." Ask yourself, "Who sent the memo?" In the first rewrite, the doer of the sending is in front of the verb. In the second rewrite, the verb is changed. The unit managers are now the doers of the verb to receive. Ask yourself, "Who received the memo?"

2. Pharmacy staff must send a copy of each prescription back to the unit with the drug.

3. The representative from Rehabilitation Therapy should prepare the agenda for the meeting.

4. Someone left the purchasing department door unlocked; this made it possible for the delivery person to pick up the computer records by mistake when he made his rounds.

Note that this example is easy because we put in the words "by someone." But see what happens in the next example.

5. (Someone) must explain fire regulations to each new employee during orientation week.

OR

During orientation week, each new employee must attend a session with the hospital's fire marshal to learn the fire regulations.

The original sentence was taken directly from a real Well Known Hospital's orientation manual. The problem at Well Known Hospital, because passive voice is used in the original, was that no one was responsible for actually explaining the fire regulations! You cannot edit that sentence; you have to send it back to the writer and ask him or her to make it clear who is to do the explaining.

6. A flowerpot, falling from the window ledge above the door, hit the chairman of the board on the head as he entered the hospital.

In this example, the flowerpot did the action, so this rewrite is in the active voice. However, the original sentence is probably better because it makes the content more relevant. So an additional warning is needed: do not become overly dependent on rules (even our rules!). Think SMART.

COMMON ERROR: WEAK PRONOUNS AND VERBS TO BEGIN SENTENCES

Poor writers tend to rely too often on pronouns (rather than nouns) and on weak beginnings to sentences. Such writing habits take all the vitality out of a written communication. In the following example, the pronoun fails to convey the correct meaning:

Students watched as instructors demonstrated the correct method for injecting medications into an intravenous tube. This is a common technique that they will be required to practise in the laboratory.

The pronoun *this* is intended to refer to the complete sense of the preceding sentence, but on first reading the pronoun seems to refer to "tube". Furthermore, the pronoun *they* later in the sentence can refer to either "students" or "instructors".

Sentences that begin with "This is…" or "There are…"—or with similar constructions (e.g., "These were…," "There is…," "That was…")—are usually weak constructions and can be strengthened merely by editing. For example:

There was a beautiful princess who lived at the edge of the forest.

This sentence would be better written as:

A beautiful princess lived at the edge of the forest.

The solution is to use strong nouns and verbs. Watch for sentences beginning with weak constructions and change them when possible. Many weak openings can simply be eliminated, as in the example above. Always watch for a pronoun (especially *they, it,* and *this*) at the beginning of a sentence and be sure that the reference to the antecedent noun is clear. Try the following exercise.

Exercise 4.3 Weak Pronouns and Verbs to Begin Sentences

Edit the following sentences:

1. There are two things that really bother me: weak pronouns and weak constructions.

2. Once upon a time, there were three little pigs who lived with their mother at the edge of the forest.

3. There are a variety of walkers that provide support to those who are weak and have difficulty maintaining balance. Some of these have wheels, although others need to be lifted with each step.

4. The nurses at Well Known Hospital use a variety of brochures, checklists, and instruction sheets to help patients learn postoperative techniques. They find the brochures are helpful and often use them to make notes about questions they need to discuss with other caregivers.

COMMENTS ON EXERCISE 4.3 WEAK PRONOUNS AND VERBS TO BEGIN SENTENCES

Following are some ways to edit and improve the sentences:

1. Two things really bother me: weak pronouns and weak constructions.

2. Once upon a time, three little pigs lived with their mother at the edge of the forest.

3. A variety of walkers provide support to those who are weak and have difficulty maintaining balance. Some walkers have wheels, although others need to be lifted with each step.

4. Nurses at Well Known Hospital use a variety of brochures, checklists, and instruction sheets to help patients learn postoperative techniques. The patients find the brochures helpful and often use them to make notes about questions they need to discuss with other caregivers.

Remember that this point is important in *written* communications. In *oral* presentations (a different route), good speakers often form a sentence with a weak beginning so that the emphasis comes at the end, when tone of voice can stress the point for listeners' ears. You probably remember that many fairy tales or children's stories prepared for reading aloud start with "Once upon a time, there was...."

COMMON ERROR: LONG, COMPLICATED, OR INAPPROPRIATE WORDS

Short, clear, simple, direct words are better than long, complex ones that may confuse, tire, or hinder the reader. In informational writing, simple words have more impact than complex ones. Everyday words are easier for the reader to understand. Complex words are often jargon (also sometimes called gobbledygook, bafflegab, officialese, or newspeak). Jargon is a derogatory term; it applies when you write "utilize" for "use" or "debark," "deplane," or "off-load" instead of "get off" or "leave." Slang (e.g., "dude"), foreign terms (e.g., "a priori," "au courant"), and outdated words (e.g., "whilst," "amongst") can also be included in this category of inappropriate terms.

Note that jargon does not mean professional terms—unless, of course, they are unsuited to your receivers. For example, "Are you suffering from an acute upper gastrointestinal tract inflammation?" is inappropriate when you want to ask a seven-year-old child "Do you have a tummy ache?" On the other hand, it would be entirely appropriate to write in the nurse's notes, "The child shows symptoms of an acute upper GI inflammation." When you, a caregiver, are writing for colleagues or other health care professionals, you must use the appropriate words. However, it is wrong when you use words only to mystify or impress or when you use terms to disorient or confound.

Often, jargon reflects popular words used in the media and, especially, in advertising, but health care has its jargon, too. Examples include "hospitalize," "operationalize," "bedrest patients," "maximize," "paradigms," "therapeutic milieu," and "conceptual frameworks." We are not saying that you should never use these words, but think SMART. Sometimes you (source) may want to baffle or buffalo your readers (audience), as some politicians frequently do! Perhaps, in some situations, you want to use big words to impress, but you must also consider the impact they may have on the reader. If an instructor feels that you are using terms only to sound impressive, he or she may start looking into your sentences carefully for errors. Another problem is that misuse of words—and it is easy to misuse complicated terms—always fails to impress. When possible, stick to strong, clear, accurate, basic English. Try the following exercise.

Exercise 4.4 Long, Complicated, or Inappropriate Words

Practise simplifying your language by giving shorter or easier equivalents for the words and phrases listed below:

utilize	achieve
attempt	ascertain
numerous	terminate
demonstrate	consult
purchase	reside
modification	explicit
subsequent	initial
accumulate	remainder
obliterate	indemnify
voluminous	endeavour
for the reason that	
her personal physician	
he totally lacked the ability to	

List three jargon terms or complex words that particularly bother you; then give their simpler equivalents.

1.

2.

3.

COMMENTS ON EXERCISE 4.4 LONG, COMPLICATED, OR INAPPROPRIATE WORDS

Following are some common substitutions. Note the word *indemnify*. You should also check a dictionary for all the meanings before you substitute a word. Take great care when you use the thesaurus tool on your computer. Be sure you appreciate all shades of meaning before you change words.

utilize	use
achieve	get, gain
attempt	try
ascertain	make sure
numerous	many
terminate	end, fire
demonstrate	show
consult	ask
purchase	buy
reside	live
modification	change
explicit	clear
subsequent	next
initial	first
accumulate	gather, get
remainder	rest
obliterate	erase, rub out
indemnify	repay
voluminous	big, large, full
endeavour	try
for the reason that	because
her personal physician	her doctor
he totally lacked the ability to	he could not

Four words that bother many instructors are "impact" used as a verb (use "affect"); "penultimate," which is almost always used incorrectly (it means *second to last*); "hopefully," which is almost always misused (leave it out); and "irregardless" (there is no such word).

Note that you cannot always substitute. In the list above, "voluminous" does not *mean* the same thing as "big," "full," or "large"; in use, it gives the reader a sense that the noun described has many folds and a great volume of material. In a way, voluminous implies all three of the shorter words. However, you are using jargon if you use "voluminous" to impress your reader or listener when "full" would do. Sometimes, you deliberately try to impress your audience with big words. Such use is still jargon—but it may be acceptable in that instance. But such use does not usually work with instructors.

COMMON ERROR: LACK OF AGREEMENT OF TERMS

Lack of agreement of terms within a sentence most commonly occurs when the writer uses a singular noun and a plural verb (or vice versa), or a singular noun and a plural pronoun (or vice versa), or a singular pronoun followed by a plural pronoun (or vice versa). Whole chapters have been written on this problem in grammar textbooks.

Look at the sentences below, which should give you some idea of this problem:

- The data is collected by questionnaire. ("Data" is a plural noun, so you need to write "The data are collected....")
- The doctors always enters the hospital through the side door. (Plural noun subject with a singular verb.)
- The nurse should take care to avoid sexist language in their quarterly reports. ("Nurse" is a singular noun; thus, the pronoun "their" should be singular ["his or her"], or, even better, the noun should be changed to a plural form.)

These three examples illustrate the most common problems with lack of agreement in sentences in student papers. Usually, you make these simple errors because you are concentrating on creating the content in the first (or second) draft. You start the sentence one way and then change your mind about the wording halfway through. Unfortunately, if you do not correct the sentence later, it will be grammatically incorrect. In the editing stage, you need to read your paper carefully to pick up such errors so that they do not appear in the final version. These errors may also represent typos rather than poor grammar, but your audience does not know that. If you make too many such errors in assignments, your instructors will get a poor impression of your abilities. You may think that such errors do not occur often, but instructors find them in about 25% of papers.

Watch for these problems when you edit. Reading your paper aloud during the final draft—as if you were reading it to someone—often helps you to spot these errors. Try the following exercise.

Exercise 4.5 Lack of Agreement of Terms

Correct the following sentences:

1. Everyone should bring a writing pad to their next class.

2. Marjorie and Lily, after spending the afternoon in classes, plans to spend the evening with their husbands.

3. The patient needs to sign a surgical consent form before the operation; if this criteria is not met, legal problems may arise.

4. For patients with autoimmune disorders, even a minor infection, such as sinusitis or flu, prove dangerous.

5. Spread of cancer cells by diffusion are prevalent in serous cavities such as the abdomen or pleura.

6. Careless disposal of needles and sharp instruments often result in injuries to hospital staff.

COMMENTS ON EXERCISE 4.5 LACK OF AGREEMENT OF TERMS

There are various ways to correct the sentences. Here are some:

1. Every<u>one</u> (singular) should bring a writing pad to the next class.

   OR

   Every<u>one</u> should bring a writing pad to his or her next class.

2. Marjorie and Lily, after spending the afternoon in classes, <u>plan</u> to spend the evening with their husbands.

3. The patient needs to sign a surgical consent form before the operation; if this <u>criterion</u> is not met, legal problems may arise. (The word *criteria,* like *data,* is plural.)

4. For patients with autoimmune disorders, even a minor infection, such as sinusitis or flu, <u>proves</u> dangerous.

   OR

   For patients with autoimmune disorders, even minor <u>infections</u>, such as sinusitis or flu, prove dangerous.

5. Spread of cancer cells by diffusion <u>is</u> prevalent in serous cavities such as the abdomen or pleura.

6. Careless disposal of needles and sharp instruments often <u>results</u> in injuries to hospital staff.

COMMON ERROR: LACK OF PARALLEL STRUCTURE

One of the most common errors in sentence structure is a failure to keep all elements that perform the same purpose within the sentence *in the same form* (i.e., *parallel*). This error is so common that grammar teachers use a symbol—//ism—to indicate faulty parallelism in a student paper.

Parallel structure allows readers to follow a list of items within the sentence clearly and quickly. Faulty parallel structure confuses and annoys the reader. For example, the following sentence indicates a lack of parallel structure:

Wrong: Mary likes swimming, golfing, and to play tennis.

The sentence lists three things that are objects of the verb *likes*—but the three things are not given in the same grammatical form. The first two ("swimming," "golfing") are gerunds, but the last one ("to play") is an infinitive verb. To be correct, they should have the same (parallel) form. When they do not, the reader does a double take and has to reread the sentence.

Correct: Mary likes swimming, golfing, and playing tennis.
Correct: Mary likes to swim, golf, and play tennis.
Correct: Mary likes to swim, to golf, and to play tennis.

Sometimes errors in parallel structure occur in the words you use to introduce a series of sentences, as in "First,…," "Secondly,…," "Third,…"; to be parallel, these words should be "first," "second," "third," or "firstly," "secondly," "thirdly." Be alert to this problem when you are doing lists (as in job descriptions). Reading aloud often alerts you to this problem.

The following two common (but simple) examples illustrate lack of parallel structure and the ways in which the sentences can be corrected:

Wrong: The lottery winner liked his new computer, his new car, and new swimming pool.
Correct: The lottery winner liked his new computer, his new car, and his new swimming pool.
Correct: The lottery winner liked his new computer, new car, and new swimming pool.
Correct: The lottery winner liked his new computer, car, and swimming pool.

Note that repetition of words may be helpful to the reader, and the first two correct examples may be easier to read than the last one. Repetition, whether explicit or implicit, provides a similarity of structure so that the reader knows what is happening.

Wrong: Mary was both required to give the intravenous drugs and to make the patient comfortable.

Correct: Mary was required both to give the intravenous drugs and to make the patient comfortable.

Correct: Mary was required to both give the intravenous drugs and make the patient comfortable.

Parallel structure sometimes requires you to understand and use common correlative constructions, such as "both... and," or "not only... but also," or "neither... nor." As you will recall from your grade school days, these constructions are bound to one another.

Wrong: Frank was required not only to give the intravenous drugs but to make the patient comfortable.

Correct: Frank was required not only to give the intravenous drugs but also to make the patient comfortable.

Sometimes a sentence can get complex and require two sets of parallel structure, as in the following example:

Wrong: I will examine context of instruction, subject matter, resources, teacher and learner characteristics and objectives, then end with a brief summary.

The two main parts of the sentence ("I will examine... then end...") need the conjunction *and*. However, the list is also complex, so the reader can only guess its meaning. The following are possible correct constructions:

Correct: I will examine context of instruction, subject matter, resources, and teacher and learner characteristics and objectives, and then end with a brief summary.

Correct: I will examine context of instruction, subject matter, resources, teacher characteristics, learner characteristics, teacher objectives, and learner objectives, and then end with a brief summary.

Note that the "extra" comma before "and" in a series (discussed in Chapter 1) makes the list clearer.

The following is another example of the lack of parallel structure:

Wrong: The objectives of the course are to learn to: identify common mistakes in language; learn to set up a manuscript properly; accurately edit papers; and familiarity with spelling styles.

Correct: The objectives of the course are to learn to identify common mistakes in language, set up a manuscript properly, edit papers accurately, and become familiar with spelling styles.

Exercise 4.6 gives a few more examples of problems with parallel structure. If they do not help you to understand parallel structure, then refer to a good grammar resource.

Exercise 4.6 Lack of Parallel Structure

1. The nurse arranged a physical examination, advised the patient about better nutrition, and then she told him how to change the dressing.

2. You either should go to the doctor's office or go to the hospital's emergency room.

3. Wet bed linen should be changed immediately because dry linen helps to prevent skin irritation and promoting psychological well-being.

4. Interventions for metabolic acidosis include recording of fluid intake and output; administration of alkaline solutions, sodium bicarbonate kept on hand for emergency use; and safety precautions if the patient is restless, confused, or convulsing.

5. Students pass the course, either by writing a paper or making a video, and presenting it to the class.

COMMENTS ON EXERCISE 4.6 LACK OF PARALLEL STRUCTURE

1. The nurse <u>arranged</u> a physical examination, <u>advised</u> the patient about better nutrition, and <u>told</u> him how to change the dressing.

2. You <u>either should</u> go to the doctor's office <u>or should</u> go to the hospital's emergency room.

OR

<u>Either go</u> to the doctor's office <u>or go</u> to the hospital's emergency room.

OR

You should go <u>either to</u> the doctor's office <u>or to</u> the hospital's emergency room.

3. Wet bed linen should be changed immediately because dry linen helps <u>to prevent</u> skin irritation and <u>to promote</u> psychological well-being.

OR

Wet bed linen should be changed immediately because dry linen helps <u>prevent</u> skin irritation and <u>promote</u> psychological well-being.

4. Interventions for metabolic acidosis include <u>recording</u> fluid intake and output; <u>administering</u> alkaline solutions as ordered; <u>having</u> sodium bicarbonate on hand for emergency use; and <u>implementing</u> safety precautions if the patient is restless, confused, or convulsing.

5. Students pass the course <u>either by</u> writing a paper <u>or by</u> making a video and presenting it to the class.

COMMON ERROR: MISUSED WORDS

Good writers generally have good vocabularies. They know a large number of words and select the most accurate one to convey meaning clearly and succinctly. For example, a good writer would know (or look up in a dictionary) the difference between a dock, a pier, and a wharf. The primary meaning for "dock" is the area of water next to a wharf or pier; a "pier" is a structure that projects out into the water from the shore; a "wharf" is a platform built along the shore (i.e., parallel to the shore). You can take a walk along a wharf, but beware if someone advises you to "Take a long walk on a short pier" or to "Go walk on a dock."

As well, good writers have learned to distinguish between homonyms (words that sound the same but have different meanings), such as "rose" (past tense of the verb *rise*) and "rose" (the flower) or "hanger" (on which you hang clothes) and "hangar" (in which you put a plane). You are expected to have learned these differences before you were admitted to a college or university. However, almost every writer has some problems with misusing words; once you know what they are, you can resolve them or avoid them. Here are 12 words or phrases frequently misused in students' papers, with some advice on how to fix them during the editing and polishing stages.

It's Versus Its

A shocking number of writers have a problem with *its* and *it's*. The following example is correct: "Nursing has its problems, but usually it's wonderful to care for patients." The word *its* is a possessive pronoun; the word *it's* is a contraction of "it is" (or, occasionally, of "it has"). Many students complain that it seems odd (or illogical) that the possessive pronoun does not take an apostrophe, as in "nursing's problems," "boy's book," or "John's dog." However, in "his book" or "the dog is hers," there are no apostrophes. You need to think of the possessive pronoun *its* as being like *his* or *hers*.

You can also use another rule. You should avoid contractions in formal writing (and you can also avoid many of them in informal writing without any problem). Therefore, if you are polishing your paper, check each time you have *its* or *it's*. If you can substitute "it is" or "it has," make the substitution and avoid the contraction. If you cannot substitute "it is" (or "it has"), use *its* (with no apostrophe). In other words, the word *it's* (with the apostrophe) would never appear in your paper! Of course, if the contraction is within a quotation from another source, you need to leave it; just be certain that you have copied it correctly.

Please note that there is no such word as *its'*.

Which Versus That

An old pun says "Instructors are 'which-hunters'—because they so often cross out *which* and substitute *that*." The two words have different meanings; both are pronouns, but *that* is restrictive or defining, and *which* is nonrestrictive or nondefining. In conversations (one route), *which* is frequently substituted for *that,* but the meaning is made clear from the way in which the speaker pauses—or fails to pause—within the sentence or from inflections in the voice. In written communications (another route), the words themselves, aided by punctuation, must convey the meaning. So, because the two words have different meanings, good writers need to know when to use *which* and when to use *that*. Consider these examples:

- The pharmacy, which is on the first floor, is closed on Sunday.
- The pharmacy which is on the first floor is closed on Sunday.
- The pharmacy that is on the first floor is closed on Sunday.

The first sentence says that there is only one pharmacy in the hospital and that it is closed on Sunday. In the second example, the meaning is not clear, but without the commas, most editors would assume *which* should be *that* and make the substitution. The third sentence implies that there may be more than one pharmacy, but the restrictive clause adds defining information; it means that the one on the first floor is closed on Sunday.

The third example can be rewritten in a way that would make the sentence shorter but just as clear:

- The first-floor pharmacy is closed on Sunday.

One good way to determine when you should use *which* is to read the sentence and see if it makes sense if you omit the nonrestrictive *which* clause. If the sentence makes sense without the clause, then use *which*, but be sure to add commas around the clause to make it completely clear to your readers. If you cannot omit the clause, then change the *which* to *that*. In other words, be your own which-hunter.

While (When It Should Be *Although, But,* or *Whereas*)

Many students use the word *while* incorrectly when they should use *although* or *but* or *whereas*. The error is simple to correct. The noun *while* means "time" (as in "for a while"). When *while* is used as a subordinating conjunction (i.e., when it ties another clause into the sentence), it still has a connotation of "time" and usually means "at the same time as." The old saying "Nero fiddled while Rome burned" is accepted as correct; "Nero fiddled while I played the piano" is correct only if I know another Nero and we are doing a duet! A good writer therefore uses *while* only when it has a timely meaning. Note the differences in meaning in the following examples:

- While I gave the medications, the doctor wrote the orders.
- Although I gave the medications, the doctor wrote the orders.
- The doctor wrote the orders while I gave the medications.
- The doctor wrote the orders, but I gave the medications.
- The doctor wrote the orders, whereas I gave the medications.

It is worth your while to learn the distinctions between *while* and *although*, *whereas*, and *but*.

Due to (When It Should Be *Because of*)

The word *due* is an adjective, not a conjunction, and the sentence must contain a noun to which *due* applies. Misuse of the phrase *due to* bothers many readers, although its use in conversation and informal writing is becoming more acceptable. Can you appreciate the differences below?

Correct:	The cheque is due to arrive in the mail.
Correct:	Her late arrival was due to the snowy weather. (*But this sentence is clumsy and could be rewritten!*)
Wrong:	Due to the snow, she was late.

If you do not understand why the first two are correct, you need to watch for this phrase when you are editing your final drafts. Look carefully at the sentence in which the phrase is used; if you can substitute *because of* for *due to*, then do so!

Feel (When You Mean *Believe*)

In most dictionaries, the primary definitions for the word *feel* relate to "touch" rather than to "sense" or "consider." Good writers thus tend to restrict the use of *feel* to the primary meanings.

Correct:	Feel the texture of his skin.
Correct:	She feels her way across the darkened room.
Wrong:	I feel this woman is ready to go to the delivery room.
Correct:	I believe (or think) this woman is ready to go to the delivery room.

Majority and Most

The word *majority* is also commonly misused in conversation and in many news stories; students tend to use it unthinkingly in formal assignments. *Majority* means the larger (of two) and thus means "more than half" or "50% plus one" or "the greater part." You cannot have "a 40% majority"; in this instance, the word should be "plurality" (or you could say "won with 40% of the votes"). The same distinctions apply to the word *most* in good writing; be sure that you mean "more than half" when you use it. Also weigh the use of *many* (as in "Many patients..."). Try to be specific when you use these words.

Between Versus Among

In grade school, you were taught the difference between these two words. *Between* relates to *two* people or things; *among* relates to *more than two*. You and I might keep a secret between us, but, according to the old adage, it becomes more difficult to keep something secret among three or more!

Affect Versus Effect

Affect is usually the verb; *effect* is usually the noun (although *affect* is occasionally used as a noun in psychology).

> *Correct:* Does a high pollen count *affect* you? What *effect* does it have?

Simply knowing that these terms commonly create problems allows you to check their use. If you have a problem with them, then avoid using them by substituting other words. For example, if you have a problem knowing whether to use *choose* or *chose*, substitute the word *select*.

To, Too, and Two

Many people never have a problem with these three homonyms, but studies show that their misuse is one of the three most common problems in business writing. (*It's* versus *its* is the most common.) If these words are problems for you, then consult a good dictionary until you finally achieve an understanding of them.

There Versus Their

The third most common error in business writing is the interchange of these two pronouns. The word *their* is a personal pronoun from the same family as *they*; *there* is similar to *this* or *that*. Consult a good grammar resource if you have problems with this pair.

Literally

Literally implies exact, precise, or actual, but has become common hyperbole in informal use to exaggerate, dramatise, or overstate. If you write "He literally won the race by a mile," you are probably exaggerating and mean that he won it by a good margin. "I literally tore my hair out over this assignment" means that you now are bald. (Some instructors believe that the word *actually* is even worse!) Avoid *literally*.

Peak Versus Peek Versus Pique

These three words sound the same but have very different meanings. A *peek* is a glance at something. A mountain tip is the *peak* and to *pique* means to capture your curiosity or interest.

Correct: I took a peek at the mountain peak and it piqued my interest.

Exercise 4.7 Misused Words

This exercise illustrates a few more of these problems and gives you a chance to assess your vocabulary.

Choose the right word in each of the following options:

1. The administrator said it was a matter of (principal, principle) with her to pay only the (principal, principle) on the loan and not the interest.

2. Joan and Mary (alternately, alternatively) checked Mrs. Green's intravenous line and monitored Mr. Smith's blood pressure and pulse.

3. Tim thought it more (discreet, discrete) to wait until he was asked for help rather than (flaunt, flout) his superior strength.

4. The drug had some (adverse, averse) side effects, causing the patient to break out in a rash.

5. Rani (lead, led) the way down the corridor.

6. She gave the report to Grace and (I, me, myself).

7. She expects to be promoted (some time, sometime) soon.

COMMENTS ON EXERCISE 4.7 MISUSED WORDS

The sentences should read as follows:

1. The administrator said it was a matter of principle with her to pay only the principal on the loan and not the interest.
   Principle *means a rule of conduct or a basic truth;* principal *in this usage means the amount borrowed, as opposed to the interest on it but can also mean most important or main or head of a school.*

2. Joan and Mary alternately checked Mrs. Green's intravenous line and monitored Mr. Smith's blood pressure and pulse.
   Alternately *means by turns;* alternatively *means choice; it might be simpler and clearer to say "Joan and Mary took turns checking Mrs. Green's intravenous line and monitoring Mr. Smith's blood pressure and pulse."*

3. Tim thought it more discreet to wait until he was asked for help rather than flaunt his superior strength.
Discreet *means tactful or prudent and implies using good judgement in conduct;* discrete *means separate or distinct;* flaunt *means to display blatantly, to show off;* flout *means to show contempt or scorn.*

4. The drug had some adverse side effects, causing the patient to break out in a rash.
Adverse *means harmful or unfavourable;* averse *means opposed or reluctant.*

5. Rani led the way down the corridor.
Lead, *pronounced to rhyme with* bead, *is the present tense of the verb* to lead *and is pronounced to rhyme with* red *only when it is used as a noun to indicate the chemical element.*

6. She gave the report to Grace and me.

7. Either is correct, although sometime, an adverb meaning at an indefinite point of time, is more common in North America.

COMMON ERROR: BIASED LANGUAGE

In recent years, good writers have had to be conscious of replacing biased language with inclusive language. Biased language represents stereotypes that unintentionally creep into writing and that may offend or even insult readers. Common biases usually represent sexist language or deal with cultural, religious, racial, or occupational terms. Biases can also apply to age categories (e.g., elderly, seniors, millennials).

Health professional students also need to be aware of biases in terms used to describe disabilities and other health-related categories.

Avoiding biased language is more than just being politically correct; good use of language can promote social well-being and help you and others to have better self-esteem. If you refer to a patient with diabetes as "a diabetic" or to a child with epilepsy as "an epileptic," you can sound as if you are using a judgemental label. If you practise avoiding biased terms in your writing, then you will also be more aware of them in oral communication. The American Psychological Association's style manuals contain an excellent review of the challenges and how to write using bias-free language. For example, to avoid sexist sentences, you could change a sentence to use plurals (*they* and *their*); substitute an article (*a, an,* or *the*) for the pronoun (*his, her, hers*); use the acceptable *his/her* alternative; or even, occasionally, omit the pronoun altogether.

Perhaps because 92.2% of nurses (Canadian Nurses Association, 2016) are female, female nursing students tend to make more mistakes with sexist language than other university students. Such habits are hard to break. Most female nurses tend to write "The nurse must be aware of the needs of all her patients." The usually accepted alternatives for the sentence above are "The nurse must be aware of the needs of all his or her patients" or, preferably, "Nurses must be aware of the needs of all their patients."

Whole books have been written on sexist language and how to avoid it, such as the original classic *Handbook of Nonsexist Writing*, by Miller and Swift (1980), which was based on earlier research. Sexist language, like other forms of sexism, hurts. Nurses, because most of them are female, should understand the stigma of sexism and avoid using sexist language. Thus, you would write "Nurses are concerned about their work environments" rather than "The nurse is concerned about his or her work environment." As well, use of the plural also helps you to avoid the "everynurse syndrome"—writing as if just one "supernurse" were involved. Furthermore, colleges and universities have taken strong stands against sexist language and have advised all faculty members to be alert to this problem. Your instructors will likely notice, comment, and maybe take off marks if you refer to any group of individuals exclusively as one gender.

As well as sexist language, this rule to avoid biases applies to other stereotypes and biases (race, colour, occupation, age, gender) where identifiers or "labels" are often given to groups (e.g., First Nations versus Indian, Indigenous people, Natives, Aboriginals, or Amerinds; Black versus African American or People of Color; Inuit versus Eskimo). APA advises that groups often make their own decisions about their preferences on what they wish to be called, although this may change over time and even within a group, which makes this a highly complex issue. Essentially, you need to recognize your unconscious usage, reflect on your language, and respect the individual and group.

The following exercise gives you some practice in noticing, editing, and avoiding biased language. Being aware of this problem will help you avoid it.

Exercise 4.8 Biased Language

PART A

The sentences below use biased terms. Try editing or rewriting them to avoid sexist terminology.

1. The head nurse should ensure that her nursing staff attend CPR drills once a year.

2. When an anaesthetist makes his rounds the evening before surgery, he needs to check with the evening admitting clerk to see if she has the list for day surgery.

3. Every student at Pennsylvania State University has his name entered in the main database.

4. To be admitted to the unit, a handicapped child must be able to dress and feed himself.

5. Dr. Alice Baumgart, past president of CNA, has been named chairman of the HEAL Committee.

6. When the new wing opens, the manpower needs of the hospital will increase 10%.

7. The telephone repairman removed the manhole cover so that he had easier access to the lines.

8. The man and his wife were upset when they found the flat tire.

PART B

Following are some common words that are suitable if you are referring to one individual and the sex is known, but that are sexist when the individual is not known. Try to supply a term that would be an acceptable nonsexist alternative.

waiter, waitress
alderman
spokesman, spokeswoman
steward, stewardess
mailman
weatherman, weather girl
fireman
poet, poetess
male nurse or female doctor

COMMENTS ON EXERCISE 4.8 BIASED LANGUAGE

PART A

You can fix sexist writing several ways. The following examples should help you to begin thinking about the appropriate use of words:

1. The head nurse should ensure that the nursing staff attend CPR drills once a year. (*OR* Head nurses should ensure that nursing staff….)

2. When the anaesthetist makes rounds the evening before surgery, he or she needs to check with the evening admitting clerk to see if the day surgery list is ready.

3. Every student at Pennsylvania State University has his or her name entered in the main database. (*OR* Students at Pennsylvania State University have their names….)

4. To be admitted to the unit, children with disabilities must be able to eat and get dressed without help. (*This version avoids the tiresome "himself or herself" and it uses the more acceptable term "disabilities" rather than "handicaps".*)

5. Dr. Alice Baumgart, past president of CNA, has been named chair of the HEAL Committee. (*OR*… named to chair the HEAL Committee.)

6. When the new wing opens, the workforce needs of the hospital will increase 10%. (*OR*… the personnel needs….)

7. The telephone repairer removed the utility-hole cover so that access to the lines was easier.

8. The husband and wife were upset when they found the flat tire. (*OR* The man and woman were upset….*) (Some readers find the phrase "man and his wife" offensive because it suggests that the woman is defined in a possessive relationship. The parallel structure of "man and woman" or "husband and wife" is preferred.*)

PART B

Following are some acceptable nonsexist alternatives:

waiter, waitress	server, waiter (*"waiter" is often recommended for both*)
alderman	councillor (*"councillor" has been officially adopted by many city and municipal councils*)
spokesman, spokeswoman	representative (*"spokesperson" may be acceptable, depending on your audience*)
steward, stewardess	flight attendant (*for unions, "steward" is used for both sexes; "steward" is also used for both sexes on ships*)

mailman	mail carrier
weatherman, weather girl	weather forecaster
fireman	firefighter *("stoker" is used for trains and ships)*
poet, poetess	poet *("poet" is recommended for both sexes)*
male nurse or female doctor	*just use "nurse" or "doctor," unless you are doing an assignment dealing, for example, with comparison of statistics*

COMMON ERROR: UNNECESSARY WORDS

You should always edit out unnecessary words, leaving sentences tighter, crisper, clearer, and easier to read. In your first draft, you may write a sentence such as the following:

> An example of this problem is the fact that fever patients need increased rest and increased fluid intake.

During editing, you could rewrite the sentence as follows:

> For example, fever patients need increased rest and increased fluids.

Most grammar books contain long lists of wordy phrases. Often a single word can be substituted or the phrase omitted altogether. The following are just a few examples of phrases that could be pared down:

- in order to (*to*)
- at the present time (*now*)
- at this point in time (*now*)
- the reason why (*the reason*)
- for the reason that (*because, since*)
- in the event that (*if*)
- are of the opinion that (*believe*)
- consensus of opinion (*consensus*)

Please watch for *in order to*; if you cannot substitute *to*, then the sentence may have a more serious problem!

Speakers (especially politicians responding to questions from journalists) tend to use long, unnecessary opening phrases to give themselves time to get their thoughts in order. Writers can organize their thoughts before they write and then edit so that readers can gain the essential message more easily. Watch for these phrases:

- It goes without saying that... (Then do not say it!)
- It is interesting to note that... (Is the rest of your paper not interesting?)

The word *the* is a special example. Many writers tend to overuse *the.* Obviously, sometimes you need to use *the,* or your sentence will be unclear or ungrammatical. Do read over your sentences, however, and see if you can remove this little word. Look at the following examples:

- The staff at the Smithview Hospital set up the additional beds in the hallways when the ambulances began arriving with the victims from the air crash.
- Staff at Smithview Hospital set up additional beds in hallways when ambulances began arriving with victims from the air crash.

In the second version, six of seven *the*'s were removed. The sentence still makes the same point, but it is much easier to read. When shining up your final drafts, look carefully for such extra words and cross them out. After a couple of years of practice, you will not even put them in!

Clichés are worn-out phrases that have been used too often. Originally, these phrases created images that sparked a reader's imagination. When they become commonplace, they no longer do that, and you need to weigh their use carefully. Either come up with a more exciting descriptive phrase that will make your paper memorable or leave out the cliché entirely. Some of the more common clichés found in student papers include the following:

- the bottom line
- quick as lightning
- good as gold
- the whole can of worms
- pretty as a picture
- quiet as a church mouse

Clichés indicate that you are a lazy writer. Avoid worn-out phrases and be original in your expressions.

Also avoid lazy words that creep into your writing but fail to make any impact on readers. In writing workshops that preceded this book, participants were asked to stand up, place the left hand over the heart, raise the right hand, and take the following pledge:

> I solemnly swear that I shall never use, in my writing, that terrible, four-letter word *very*.

Participants had a lot of trouble with that final word; they could not understand why *very* was singled out for a pledge. However, even years later, individuals would comment that they have become better writers because they took that pledge and that they still feel guilty whenever they are tempted to write *very*. This may seem simplistic, but if you, too, follow this rule, your writing will improve. If you take the pledge to give up *very*, you will be forced to think about your vocabulary. And that means you will take a big step on the road to improvement in your writing.

Very is the worst of a long list of lazy words that weaken your writing. Other extraneous words include *quite, rather, some, lots, many,* and *few.* Think about these words for a minute. How much smaller than small is very small or rather small? If you mean tiny, minute, microscopic, or infinitesimal, then use one of those words—or, in writing, just use *small* on its own. How big is very big? Gigantic, enormous, huge, 298 pounds, six foot seven inches, 32 billion? When you are speaking, you can use body language (e.g., raise your eyebrows) and tones of voice (e.g., drawl the word *very*) to convey meaning. In your writing, however, *very* just signals that the following word was not strong enough on its own. Substituting the word *extremely* is no better; you have just used a bigger word to get around the real problem.

Think, as well, about misuse of *very*. If you write, "She was a very honest nutritionist," does that imply there are degrees of honesty?

The correct solution is to use strong, accurate, and descriptive nouns, adjectives, and verbs. When you go over your paper during the editing or polishing phase, look for lazy words. To practise, try the following exercise.

Exercise 4.9 Unnecessary Words

Look over the following sentences and cross out lazy words that add nothing to the paragraph:

1. Physiotherapists very often neglect to mention quite obvious hazards when they are teaching patients to walk with a cane.

2. The implementation of these findings has been very slow.

3. In order to write well, remove all extraneous and superfluous words.

4. The day was extremely frigid. Rather than spend quite a long time dressing all the residents in their outdoor clothes to take them out for some exercise, the recreational therapists decided to hold a dance in the foyer.

COMMENTS ON EXERCISE 4.9 UNNECESSARY WORDS

This exercise was set up to help you find unnecessary words; almost all the sentences could be rewritten to make them stronger.

1. Physiotherapists ~~very~~ often neglect to mention ~~quite~~ obvious hazards when they are teaching patients to walk with a cane.

2. ~~The~~ implementation of these findings has been ~~very~~ slow.

3. ~~In order~~ to write well, remove ~~all extraneous and~~ superfluous words.

4. The day was ~~extremely~~ frigid. Rather than spend ~~quite~~ a long time dressing ~~all the~~ residents in ~~their~~ outdoor clothes to take them out for ~~some~~ exercise, ~~the~~ recreational therapists decided to hold a dance in the foyer.

COMMON ERROR: INCONSISTENCIES IN SPELLING, PUNCTUATION, AND CAPITALIZATION

During the editing and polishing phases, you should review punctuation, spelling, and capitalization. You should look especially for inconsistencies.

Problems related to inconsistencies in spelling style were discussed in Chapter 1, and this is a good time to review them. While creating your message, you may read several books and journals. If so, you may carry the style used in your readings into your paraphrases, writing "a woman in labor" on one page and "the labour and delivery room" a few pages later. Note that *judgement* and *judgment* are both correct. Which is more common in Canada? in the United States? in Britain? Which is recommended in the dictionary you use? Which is used by the spell-checker in your software program? The APA manuals recommend that you follow the spelling used in *Merriam-Webster* dictionaries, which are widely used in the United States, but many Canadian colleges and universities recommend that a *Gage* or an *Oxford* dictionary be used as a spelling guide. The publisher for our book uses the *Canadian Oxford Dictionary* (Barber, 2004), so note, for example, the spelling of the word *colour* (not *color*) would be used in the text of this book (unless we are using an example in APA style). Usually, your instructors are not dogmatic about spelling style as long as you are consistent throughout the paper.

You also need to watch the style used in punctuation, another problem area mentioned in Chapter 1. You have to decide—based on Source * Message * Audience * Route * Tone—which punctuation style to use. For example, you need to decide whether to use a comma before *and* in a series of three or more items, as in "We bought apples, oranges(,) and bananas." This is a matter of style, but in formal academic writing, the comma usually goes in before *and*. In many journals and most newspapers, this comma is omitted. The APA manuals recommend use of this comma; if you are required to use APA style, then watch for this point. You must be consistent in the way you use this comma.

In North America, periods (and most other punctuation marks) belong inside quotation marks, unless the meaning would be altered. As you create a rough draft, however, do not worry about the position. As you do the critical review in the editing and polishing stages, you should look at the position of every punctuation mark.

Use of hyphens is partly a style matter and partly a spelling matter. Furthermore, use will change over time. Would you write "Health professionals are concerned about a patient's *well-being*" (or use *wellbeing* or *well being*)? Think about the following alternatives:

- caregiver OR care-giver
- e-mail OR email (APA used to recommend the former; now both APA style and *Oxford* dictionaries use the latter)
- lifestyle OR life-style
- president elect OR president-elect
- postoperative OR post-operative (APA style recommends the former; *Oxford* dictionary, the latter)

Compound words take many styles: some are written as two words; some are joined as one word; some are hyphenated. Furthermore, some vary depending on usage in the sentence (e.g., "The lab did an occult-blood test," but "The lab tested for occult blood"). The best tool to help you with hyphens is a good dictionary. You should find out which dictionary is recommended in your program and look up the word. Remember, however, that when phrases are used in different ways, the spelling or hyphenation may change. The spell-checker on your computer may not be helpful with hyphens; for example, most spell-checkers accept both *pre-operative* and *preoperative* as correct spellings, even within the same sentence. Note the following differences in hyphen usage:

- Public health nurses give follow-up care. (Used in the adjective.)
- Public health nurses follow up clients. (Not used in the verb.)
- Instructors often use role playing in their classes. (Not used in the noun.)
- Role-playing techniques offer students opportunities to learn in nonstressful situations. (Used in the adjective.)

Most style manuals recommend using hyphenated phrases only when necessary for clarity. The usual problem is that students are not consistent and sometimes use a hyphen and then later do not use a hyphen in the same word used the same way in a sentence. Watch—and be consistent!

Another area in which students have problems concerns inconsistency with capital letters. You will face decisions every time you write. For example, if you are writing a paper outlining changes in the organization of Well Known Hospital, you might write something like the following:

> At its June *Meeting*, the *Board of Directors* of Well Known Hospital voted to replace its *Advisory Council* formerly representing *Specialty Practice Groups* with a new *Health Professionals' Forum*. The *board* decided the *forum* would allow individual professions to speak with a united voice and lead to better communication on issues such as *Liability Insurance*.

OR

> At its June *Meeting*, the *board of directors* of Well Known Hospital voted to replace its *advisory council* formerly representing *specialty practice groups* with a new *health professionals' forum*. The *Board* decided the *Forum* would allow individual professions to speak with a united voice and lead to better communication on issues such as *liability insurance*. [Note that *liability insurance* usually would not require capitals.]

In both the above passages, there are inconsistencies. You have to decide whether to use capital letters for many of the titles (an "up style") or not to use capital letters (a "down style")— except for specific names (i.e., June, Well Known Hospital). However, once that style decision is made, all subsequent use should be consistent with the determined style. But should this decision about style be yours? As noted in Chapter 1, Source * Message

* Audience * Route * Tone can affect style. In making decisions about style for formal student assignments, two important elements of the SMART way need to be considered: audience and route. Has your instructor told you, either in class or in the course syllabus, that you are required to use a certain style manual (e.g., the APA or other manual or style sheet)? If so, then you should use it.

Even if your instructor has not specified a style manual, the route itself may dictate that you use one. When you were in high school, your assignments required a certain form, but that form may not be what is required at college or university. The level of papers rises, and you are probably not well versed on the style decisions required. Style for college-level papers involves many elements!

Therefore, either of the following would be correct:

At its June *meeting*, the *Board of Directors* of Well Known Hospital voted to replace its *Advisory Council* formerly representing *Specialty Practice Groups* with a new *Health Professionals' Forum*. The *Board* decided the *Forum* would allow individual professions to speak with a united voice and lead to better communication on issues such as *liability insurance*. [This is a style favoured by public relations departments.]

OR

At its June *meeting*, the *board of directors* of Well Known Hospital voted to replace its *advisory council* formerly representing *specialty practice groups* with a new *health professionals' forum*. The *board* decided the *forum* would allow individual professions to speak with a united voice and lead to better communication on issues such as *liability insurance*. [This is the style recommended by the APA manuals.]

Exercise 4.10 gives you an opportunity to catch some inconsistencies. Try it.

Exercise 4.10 Inconsistencies in Spelling, Punctuation, and Capitalization

The following two paragraphs contain many common compound words or phrases. The paragraphs contain some repetition and some informal words, and they could certainly be edited to make the sentences stronger. However, the exercise is to get you thinking about style inconsistencies and especially rules for hyphens. Simply insert hyphens where necessary.

You should also look for inconsistencies in use of capitals and watch for a spelling mistake.

> The vicepresident (patient care) decided that it was time to upgrade her 10 year old, workworn computer system by adding up to date softwear and databases with a cloud computing service. She called a face to face meeting with the hospital's head of information technology (IT) services and the secretary from the human relations department. She preferred meetings rather than one page memos or email; as well, with a meeting she could obtain feedback.
>
> As her Staff arrived for the meeting, she thought how lucky she was to have such a hardworking group (not a donothing or clockwatcher among them). She said that her aboutface on computer replacement came when the old fashioned softwear system she had been using let two hyphens slip by her Xray vision. She said that she felt a loss of self esteem, and it was all downhill for the old fashioned system after that.

COMMENTS ON EXERCISE 4.10 INCONSISTENCIES IN SPELLING, PUNCTUATION, AND CAPITALIZATION

For the corrected version below, we put in hyphens based on the use recommended in the *Canadian Oxford Dictionary* (Barber, 2004). Other dictionaries or style manuals may recommend other usage. The only spelling error was "softwear." Although you could have elected to put all staff titles in capital letters, the use of lower case letters is preferred, is recommended in APA guidelines, and is easier to read.

> The *vice-president* (patient care) decided that it was time to upgrade her *10-year-old*, workworn computer system by adding *up-to-date software* and databases with a cloud computing service. She called a *face-to-face* meeting with the hospital's head of information technology (IT) service and the secretary from the human relations department. She preferred meetings rather than *one-page* memos or email; as well, with a meeting she could obtain feedback.
>
> As her staff arrived for the meeting, she thought how lucky she was to have such a hardworking group (not a *do-nothing* or *clock-watcher* among them). She said that her *about-face* on computer replacement came when the old-fashioned *software* system she had been using let two hyphens slip by her *X-ray* vision. She said that she felt a loss of *self-esteem*, and it was all downhill for the *old-fashioned* system after that.

COMMON ERROR: MISUSE OF i.e. AND e.g.

Do you ever have trouble deciding if you should use i.e. or e.g. in a sentence? You are not alone; mastering the correct use of these meaningful letters is challenging. The two abbreviations are not interchangeable. As well, you do not use these abbreviations except within parentheses in your formal assignments.

Both abbreviations come from Latin roots with i.e. meaning *that is* (in Latin *id est*) and e.g. meaning *for example* (in Latin *exempli gratia*). You use i.e. to explain something in different words or to add or clarify. You use e.g. to indicate to your readers that examples follow. One way to check to see if you are using i.e. correctly is to replace it with the phrase *in other words*, or *that is to say*, or *that is*. Does your sentence still make sense? If the answer is yes, then you are using i.e. appropriately. To check your use of e.g., substitute the words *for example* for the e.g. in your sentence.

> *Correct*: Pablo likes to eat breakfast in the sunniest location in the kitchen (i.e., the nook). (The sentence would make sense if you substitute *in other words*, or *that is to say*, or *that is* for i.e.).
>
> *Correct*: Aisha was prescribed many medications (e.g., antidepressants, analgesics, anticoagulants). (The sentence would make sense if you substitute *for example* for e.g.).

Deciding when to use e.g. and when to use i.e. is the first step in avoiding an error. Remember these abbreviations are not italicized; even though they represent Latin words, they are commonly used in English. You need a period after each letter because they are abbreviations. Most style guides require a comma after both i.e. and e.g..

Exercise 4.11 Choosing Between i.e. and e.g.

Read each sentence below and decide if the abbreviation was used correctly:

1. I travelled to Mexico last week and I packed my most colourful bathing suit (i.e., the lime green one).

2. Paul enjoyed many hobbies (e.g., polo, hunting, fishing).

3. Kelly found a coupon code to substantially reduce the cost of printer ink (i.e., 50% off).

4. Keegan grew a huge urban garden with many vegetables (i.e., corn, peas, beans).

COMMENTS ON EXERCISE 4.11 CHOOSING BETWEEN I.E. AND E.G.

1. You could substitute the phrase *that is, in other words,* or *that is to say* for the i.e. in the sentence, so i.e. is correct.

2. Polo, hunting, and fishing are examples of Paul's hobbies, so e.g. is correct.

3. You are clarifying when you say 50% off means substantially, so i.e. is correct.

4. Corn, peas, and beans are examples so e.g. (not i.e.) would be the correct abbreviation.

COMMON ERROR: POOR PARAGRAPHING

A complaint we hear from instructors is that students do not know how to use paragraphs correctly (a subject that is taught in about Grades 4 through 8). So here is a quick review about paragraphs related to academic papers.

A paragraph is a *unit* within a section of the body of your essay (paper). In your outline, you have divided the topic of your paper into three main sections (see Chapter 2 for more on outlines). Then you need to develop paragraphs within each section that explore those parts of your topic. As such, the paragraph itself should have a beginning (usually called a *topic sentence*), a middle, and an end. Generally, the paragraph deals with one thought that develops a specific line of reasoning that builds up your views on the main subject of your paper.

So, for example, if in one section of a relatively short paper you were discussing the three main types of wines (i.e., red, white, and rosé), you might use three paragraphs, one on each type. For the first sentence of the paragraph, you might write, "The most popular type of wine consumed in North America is white." You would then go on to discuss types of grapes used to make white wines and perhaps part of the winemaking process. You would continue to develop the main idea related to the topic of the paper as needed—and with consideration for the length of your finished paper. You might then start the next paragraph with the topic sentence: "The second most popular wines are the varieties of reds, ranging from fullbodied, heavy wines to consume with meats, to delicate, light reds for sipping on summer afternoons on the patio." To create a logical progression, your third paragraph should have a similar—but not boringly repetitive—topic sentence related to rosé. You may also need another paragraph (or more) in the section that would begin: "Other main groups of wines, such as ice wines and fruit wines, are making a bid for popularity." And so on.

You also need to have transitions between paragraphs. Sometimes this is done by introductory words, such as *first, second*, and *third. Also* is another valuable transition phrase, as are *furthermore, therefore, again*, and *in addition*. If you use *on the other hand,* just be sure you limit the use to two items.

Another problem with paragraphing lies in the ways citations are used within a paragraph—as will be commonplace in many of your assignments. Placing a single citation at the end of a paragraph is correct when all the items were taken from that one resource. However, instructors tell us that frequently it is obvious that more than one resource was used in the paragraph—and you will lose marks if you have not cited each resource in the appropriate place.

Paragraphs may be short or long, or even composed of only one sentence. Short paragraphs are often used for emphasis; one sentence paragraphs are rare in academic papers.

On the other hand, paragraphs that are too long are difficult to read. Instructors reiterate to us that paragraphs that go on for three or four pages are too long. So you need to be vigilant and look at your paper with a watchful eye when you are searching for common errors. A quick look at appropriate paragraphing can be seen in the sample student paper in Appendix A. Remember this advice is for formal academic papers. Other rules of style apply when you are writing dialogue and fictional stories. When you write your first novel, take a brief course on those styles.

POINTS TO REMEMBER

❏ The final review (the editing and shining steps) of your draft is important to help you detect common errors.

❏ This review can take time, which means you need to schedule it into your assignment plan.

❏ Use all your major writing tools (dictionary, style manual, grammar checker) for this review.

❏ If you have time, ask a family member, friend, or classmate to check your paper for typos and common errors.

❏ You will get much faster with practice, and what are now separate, time-consuming steps will soon become second nature. For example, you should soon stop writing *very* and start thinking about the most accurate word even as you write the first draft. You will be alert to parallel structure when you start to make a list. You will be visualizing your readers while you are drafting and therefore starting to make your language suitable to your audience.

❏ Be consistent in your spelling, capitalization, and punctuation styles.

❏ You may think that all this sounds like nit-picking. Remember, however, what nits really are. If you do not pick them out, you end up with a lousy paper!

REFERENCES

Barber, K. (Ed.). (2004). *Canadian Oxford dictionary* (2nd ed.). Don Mills, ON: Oxford University Press.

Canadian Nurses Association. (2016). *Registered nurses profile (including nurse practitioners), Canada*. Retrieved from https://cna-aiic.ca/en/nursing-practice/the-practice-of-nursing/health-human-resources/nursing-statistics/canada

Flesch, R. (1960). *How to write, speak, and think more effectively*. New York: New American Library. NOTE: The Flesch Reading Ease Formula is also available online at http://www.readabilityformulas.com/flesch-reading-ease-readability-formula.php

Miller, C., & Swift, K. (1988). *The handbook of nonsexist writing: For writers, editors and speakers* (2nd ed.). NY: Harper & Row.

5 SMART ways for specific routes

The SMART elements of communication and the steps in the writing PROCESS will work for you throughout your career. Once you have practised using them and have learned the basics related to each type of written communication, you should be able to master each new route fairly quickly. So far in this book, we have concentrated mainly on preparation of student papers and on how to use APA style. Appendix A gives you more on the fundamentals about student assignments, and an illustration of a fictional paper—one too long to include in this chapter.

This chapter goes over the fundamentals of other routes that you will meet in your career: documentation and charting; business letters; electronic communications; class presentations; résumés and curriculum vitae; reports; minutes and agendas; research papers, theses, and dissertations; and articles. If you are a beginning student, you can go directly to Appendix A but come back for all the other routes. Each one requires practice, of course, but you can learn and apply numerous details for each type; in fact, you can find at least one whole book devoted to each of the routes. But if you think SMART and draw on the basics from earlier in this book, you should adapt well to all routes.

DOCUMENTATION AND CHARTING

Health care professionals are required to document accurately any care provided; this is to meet legal and professional standards. Documentation (also referred to as charting or recording) includes electronic or written details about interactions with patients or about care provided. Documentation assists communication among health care team members, promotes safe and appropriate care, is useful for quality improvement and risk management, and facilitates evidence-informed practice. Accurate and complete patient records are essential. The saying is, "If something is not documented, it did not happen." If legal proceedings should arise related to patient care, your documentation will be considered a reflection of what occurred. It may also serve as your memory trigger if a trial is required after a long time. The importance of quality documentation cannot be overemphasized.

The following principles of excellent documentation will guide you to success with this writing route. These basics apply to both electronic and handwritten charting, although the processes may be slightly different.

Charting must be timely and include relevant information related to patient assessment, status, care interventions, and outcomes of interventions; essentially everything related to a patient's care. Aim for succinctness and clarity in your writing; resist the temptation to write a novel! If you choose to use abbreviations in your charting, check your agency policy on approved abbreviations. Timeliness should be your goal; chart your observations, actions, and interactions as soon as you are able. If you must make a late entry (a comment that is out of chronological order) indicate the actual date and time of the event. Avoid the temptation to chart anything before you do it. For example, you may plan to give a medication or treatment at a certain time, but do not chart this until you have completed it. Your plan might be disrupted, and your pre-charting would be an error.

Be objective; document what you see, hear, and do in unbiased terms. Your opinions have no place in your charting; concisely state the facts. If you are documenting something the patient said, make this clear. For example, you could write "Patient stated his pain was 8/10." Using quotes from patients is a good strategy for keeping your charting objective.

Accuracy is essential. If you applied the correct dressing but you charted it incorrectly, it is an error. Legibility is becoming less of a consideration with increased use of electronic documentation, but if you do need to document by hand, write so others can accurately read your writing. If you are using handwritten charting, make sure you only use the ink colours approved at your facility. Know the policy at your workplace for correcting charting errors. With handwritten notes the correct process is usually to strike out the mistake with a single line (so the original is still legible) and then to write "error" and your initials above the incorrect entry. Do not leave blank lines between entries or be tempted to squeeze in a line if you forgot to chart something in sequence. The main principle to keep in mind is that altering or falsifying your documentation deliberately to mislead or cover up an error is a criminal offense. Any changes made to charting must be done in a timely and honest manner.

You are responsible for charting your own observations and actions. Other health team members will document their own. The one time you may need to document another person's actions is during an emergency, such as a code scenario when you may be the designated recorder.

Many different charting and documentation systems and tools exist. Examples include flow-sheets, clinical pathways, narrative notes, and checklists. Learn how to use the system specific to your agency and only use the approved system or form. Charting practices also vary from organization to organization; when you begin work in a new facility, review the policies related to documentation as part of your orientation.

You need to take accountability and responsibility for your charting. This is usually done by signing your entries with your name and credentials, or by using a unique identifier with electronic health records. If you are charting electronically, make sure you use a strong password (changed often and never shared) to protect your unique identifier. Log off when you finish each charting session to keep your entries secure.

One special type of documentation is a report completed when an incident occurs, such as a patient fall or medication error. This is sometimes called a safety event report or an incident report. The format and name vary from facility to facility, but the main purpose is to record the facts related to the incident for use in quality improvement actions. Each organization has a process for using this document to determine factors that may have contributed to the event and to put in place strategies to prevent reoccurrence. Incident or safety reports are not part of the patient record.

BUSINESS LETTERS

You learned the fundamentals of business letters in grade school and have probably already had to write a number of business letters. For example, many health care programs require that you write a formal letter of application, which is one type of business letter. During your course, you may also need to communicate formally with your faculty or with an instructor, and you may need to use a business letter to do that.

All letters have a similar basic form. As the writer of the letter, you are the source. Even if you are sending much the same message (e.g., "I am applying for a job"), each audience (e.g., friend, personnel officer) will likely be different. Even if you are a friend of the person to whom you are sending a business letter, you treat it differently because it is not sent to just that person but may become part of the office or agency files. The main differences between a personal letter (i.e., one you would send to a friend) and a business letter are in a few rules of route and a distinct difference in tone. However, even business letters can have differences in tone, from highly formal to informal, but still remain business-like.

You can now send business letters electronically, but usually these are sent as email attachments so that they may be entered into an agency's electronic files. Digital signatures may be added and usually are acceptable, although some legal documents require encrypted signatures or that you sign, scan, and send as a PDF file.

Almost all business letters are done as if they were to be printed on 8½" × 11" stationery. If you are sending a hard copy version, the paper should be of good quality and be either a basic white or a neutral, formal colour (cream, grey, pale blue) and should have a business-size envelope (9" × 4" or 9½" × 4") that matches in colour. Letters are folded into three to fit into these envelopes. You can get coloured and printed (e.g., floral) stationery that fits into your printer, but save this fancy paper for personal letters.

Business letters generally should be typed. Some potential employers like to see your handwriting because it often reveals details about you (e.g., whether you can spell). If you write neatly and legibly, a short, handwritten letter of application that accompanies a typed résumé will probably be acceptable to most hospital or health agency personnel offices. If you are writing an application asking for several thousand dollars of funding for equipment on your unit, then you would be wise to think carefully about the formatting. If you are writing a letter of thanks to the president of the volunteers on behalf of your unit, a legible, handwritten note on hospital stationery would usually be acceptable and might convey a warmer, friendlier tone than a typed letter. If, on behalf of the staff of your unit, you are writing a letter of condolence to the family of a former patient, a sympathy card with a handwritten note might be the most appropriate route.

Basic Format of a Business Letter

As you may remember from your school days, the basic format for a business letter is as follows:

- address or letterhead
- date
- file numbers (optional)
- inside address (complete name and address of the individual and company to whom you are writing, including all details, such as postal code)
- reference line(s) (optional; may go below the salutation)
- salutation (the "Dear..." line, sometimes optional)
- body of the letter (in which you use the outline discussed in Chapter 2)
- complimentary close
- signature
- typed name (sometimes optional; e.g., it would be omitted if you use your own letterhead)
- stenographic reference (writer's or typist's initials)
- note regarding enclosures or copies

Box 5.1 shows the basic format for a relatively simple business letter. The sample is set in a style known as "flush left," which has been adopted by businesses in recent years; all new sections of the letter, including paragraphs, start at the left-hand margin. A more traditional indented style (where the date is on the right side of the page, each line in the inside address is

Sample Business Letter, Flush Left Style

Well Known Hospital
54321 Major Drive
Well Known City, BC V4Z X0O
Telephone (604) 555-1234

December 18, 2019

File: 02:30

Ms. Anne Applicant, RN
1234 Urban Ave.
Well Known City, SK S7R TK0

RE: Application for RN position

Dear Ms. Applicant

The Personnel Office has given me your letter of application. You expressed interest in a position in Extended Care, and I will have an opening at the end of January. Our unit has 46 long-term female residents, mainly elderly, but also has a few young women with severe physical and mobility limitations. I have looked over your letter and résumé, and I believe you may have the skills we need for our unit's team of nurses.

I will be holding interviews with two other possible applicants in early January. If you also would like an interview, please telephone me as soon as possible so that we can schedule a time.

The best times to reach me are weekday afternoons between 1300 and 1500 hours. Telephone the hospital number above and use extension 305.

Sincerely

Kerin Smithers, RN, BSN
Unit Care Manager
Westbrook Unit

KS/at
Copy: Personnel Office, T. K. Paterson

indented a couple of spaces, paragraphs are indented with a tab, and the closing is centred on the page) is suitable for handwritten business letters. If you type your own business letters, follow the flush left style because it is by far the easiest to set up. Various styles are recommended for spacing between sections and individual paragraphs; if you do the spacing yourself, position the letter in the centre of the page and leave double spaces between paragraphs. Many types of templates for business letters are available online.

Basic components for a business letter are given below. Some of these apply to other routes, such as memos and email messages.

Address or Letterhead

If you are writing a business letter on behalf of your employer, you would use the letterhead of the hospital, agency, or company; you are acting as a source on behalf of that agency. The letterhead contains the return address, and all mail in reply to your letter would be sent to that address. You may need to add a typed line to indicate how mail should be directed to you within the agency (e.g., name of department or unit).

You would almost never use a company letterhead and ask for a reply to be sent to you at another address (e.g., your home address), although there are a few exceptions (e.g., when you write on behalf of a club or association and wish to speed up mail delivery); you need, however, to make this point clearly in the body of the letter.

You may also need to write business letters from your home on your own behalf (e.g., to apply for a job, to write to a politician or a newspaper stating an opinion, or to ask for a correction to a bank document). In today's world of computers, you can easily develop your own letterhead, as shown in Box 5.2, and save it on your computer. Templates to help you design your own letterhead are available online, but you should choose a style appropriate for your audience. Letterheads are not difficult to design, but you need to keep SMART principles in mind as you do so. For business, the letterhead should be slightly formal; plain is generally better than fancy,

---

BOX 5.2   Sample Personal Letterhead

Glennis Zilm

306 Wood St., Black Rock, BC V4O 3V6
Telephone (604) 555-0111 Email Glennis@bol.com

---

but you can think SMART. For example, Beyoncé might select a more daring letterhead than you would choose, especially if you were writing to a public health department asking for a staff position. If you (source) weigh the message, audience, and tone, you should be able to design a personal business letterhead that is creative and suitable.

Information Before the Body of the Letter

Many people wonder whether they should write December 22, 2019 or 22 December 2019 or another version for the date of the letter. We like the former (especially for a lay audience, as shown in the sample letter), with the month spelled out, but you (source) can use the format you want. Note that some health care agencies use the international format (the latter version), and your instructors (audience) may wish you to follow that style.

A file number is only necessary in a large agency, such as a hospital, and you have to learn the method used. A file number might be used on job applications, as in the sample letter shown in Box 5.1. If you are responding to a letter that used a file number, you should quote that number in any further correspondence. For example, if Anne Applicant responded to Kerin Smithers, she would put in this line: "Your file number: 02:30."

The inside address is an essential part of a business letter and should be as complete as possible. For best results, you should always try to find the name of a person to whom to address your letter (although this information is not always available). For example, if you are writing a letter to the editor of a professional journal, you should check a recent issue to find the name of the editor. If you are sending a job application to a small hospital or agency in your area, you may want to search online for the contact information of the appropriate person. If you are writing to a large urban hospital, where there are likely several people working in the department, you could address the letter to the Personnel Office or the Human Resources Department. Remember, however, that almost any reader likes to be addressed by name.

Address the recipient by name in the salutation; thus, you do not have to use the completely out-of-date "To Whom It May Concern" or the old-fashioned "Dear Sir or Madam"; some recipients find these salutations (especially the latter) offensive. Many letter writers worry about how to word the salutation when they have only the initials of the person or have a first name for a woman but do not know whether to write "Ms.," "Mrs.," or "Miss." Our advice to these worriers is to concentrate on writing a good message in the body of the letter. Then simply think SMART about the details of the salutation. If you do find the recipient's name, also try to find out if it belongs to a Mr., Mrs., Miss, Ms., or Dr. You can also use the first name or initials with the last name if that is the way the person has signed a letter to you (e.g., "Dear Mary Jones" or "Dear M. T. Jones"). If you do not have a name, you can omit the salutation altogether and just use a reference line. (See the sample job application letter Box 5.3.)

BOX 5.3   Sample Job Application Letter

1234 Urban Street
Thunder Bay, AB T8G 0X0

June 23, 2019

Human Resources/Personnel Office
Well Known Regional Hospital
4321 Main Street
Prince George, BC V2L 0N0

RE: Application for Registered Nurse Position

My husband and I are moving to Prince George in mid-August, and I am seeking a position as a staff nurse. He will be joining the teaching staff at Prince George Elementary School.

As you will see from my résumé, I graduated in late April from the School of Nursing at Thunder Bay Community College, and I have passed my Registered Nurse exams. I am registered with the College and Association of Registered Nurses of Alberta, and I applied for registration with the College of Registered Nurses of B.C. earlier this month.

Since graduation, I have been working as a casual relief nurse at the Eagle Ridge Hospital near Thunder Bay, mainly in the Long-Term Care Units. The local hospitals do not have any openings for full-time staff, but I have been assured that my work skills are excellent, and I would be in line for a full-time position should one arise. My unit supervisors have agreed to supply letters if you require references. As well as my nursing jobs, I have worked part time as an assistant in a day care centre (12 infants).

I would like to receive information about your hospital and application forms for a possible RN position. If you expect to have an opening before mid-August and would like to discuss it with me, I can be reached by telephone at (403) 555-0137 or by email at summers@bol.com.

Sincerely

(Mrs.) Geraldine Summers, RN

The reference line usually highlights the subject of the letter (as in the example in Box 5.1). You can use "RE:" or "Re:" or "Subject:". The reference component is usually underlined, but some writers prefer to use all capital letters. A reference line might also be used to highlight something important, such as "Personal and confidential."

Some style guides for business letters suggest using the reference line to direct your letter to a person within the company, as in the following example:

Personnel Office
Well Known Hospital
54321 Major Drive
Well Known City, BC V4Z X0O

ATTENTION: Mary Jones, Personnel Officer

Dear Ms. Jones,

This kind of address might be used if you had spoken to Mary Jones on the telephone before you sent the letter but wanted it to convey the message that you were sending a general letter of application (and not writing to her personally).

Information After the Body of the Letter

The complimentary close comes immediately after the body of the letter, separated by a double space. The complimentary close most commonly used now in business letters is "Sincerely," although some companies use "Yours truly." Some complimentary closes are long outdated, such as "Your faithful servant." (And, after reading Chapter 4 in this book, you would never use "Very truly yours," would you?) If you have had a long business correspondence with a person or have come to know him or her, you might want use a more familiar close like "Best wishes."

After the complimentary close, you leave some space for your signature. For business letters to someone you do not know, you should generally avoid using nicknames or diminutives and develop a consistent signature (e.g., Marjorie Jones rather than Marj Jones). Once you know the correspondent well, you may elect to sign with the name that she or he calls you (e.g., Marj). Your courtesy title (e.g., Mrs.), your degree(s) (e.g., RN), and your title (e.g., Unit Manager) are not handwritten.

The typed signature line goes below your signature, even if the latter is legible. This line does contain the courtesy title and agency job title and may contain the specialty designation (registration or licensing) credentials and degrees. Make it clear in the typed signature how you wish to be addressed. For example, you may sign the letter "Nancy Nadon," but the typed signature might read "(Mrs.) Nancy Nadon, P.T." or "(Ms.) Nancy Nadon, PT." Whether you use periods with the initials can be your choice in a personal letter; it may depend on the route.

If you type your own letter, you do not need a stenographic reference. If someone else types your letter, he or she will put in your initials followed by his or her own.

If you are adding enclosures to the letter or sending a copy to another person or department, make a note to this effect by adding the accepted abbreviations for enclosure (enc or encl) or carbon copy (cc).

Helpful Hints for the Body of the Letter

Although we have taken a number of pages to go over the rules of the route for letters, always remember that the message in the body of the letter is the most important part. The ways to develop a good body of a letter are the same as those described in Chapters 1 through 4. First of all, think SMART.

Keep in mind who you (source) are and why you are writing. If you are writing on behalf of your employer, be aware that what you say and how you say it will reflect on your employer (and ultimately on your job). Sometimes you are writing on behalf of those who work for you.

Determine what your message is; you may even want to summarize it in the reference line so that it will be at the top of the letter. Your message should be presented in the same three-part outline that works for assignments. The opening paragraph, which should be short, is the introduction and tells the recipient what the letter is about. The body of the message is conveyed in the next paragraph or two (or more, if necessary). The final paragraph, which also should be short, is the conclusion and should sum up what you want the recipient of the letter to do. Like the conclusion to a student paper, the final paragraph or sentence will stay in the reader's mind, so it should be positive, stimulating, and creative. Depending on the importance of the letter, you may want to spend extra time on the beginning and ending as well as on the important body information in the middle. If you are writing a letter to your mother, she will likely be so delighted to hear from you that you can open with a trite remark such as "How are you? I am fine" and close with "Give my love to Dad, and ask him to send me an extra 10 dollars for a pizza." On the other hand, if you are writing a letter to graduates of your faculty of pharmacy to raise funds for a student scholarship, you should be particularly creative so that they all will read the opening, the body, and the conclusion—and then send some money!

Try to visualize the person to whom you are writing (audience) and the setting in which he or she will be reading your letter (e.g., a busy office, with 17 other similar letters on the desk). Think about the information your reader will want and try to present your message with consideration for the reader's point of view. What information does this person want or need in your letter?

Finally, consider the tone of the letter. Try to see, again in your mind's eye, the recipient of your letter as a friend (even if you are writing a letter to complain about something). This visualization exercise will usually help you to set a good tone, and you can choose words that will make a positive impression. Is your business letter to be a begging letter, a demanding letter, a whining letter, a bitter letter? Even if the message is negative, you can use a positive tone; positive reactions from your audience will likely lead to better results. For example, if you are writing to complain about a mistake, the individual who gets the letter is probably not the one who made the mistake; why antagonize this person? If you get the reader on your side, the mistake is more likely to be corrected.

After thinking SMART, go over the steps of the writing PROCESS: Plan * Research * Organize * Create * Edit * Shine * Submit! Just as with an assignment, if you take a few minutes on the "PRO" steps (plan, research, and organize) before you start to compose your letter, you will write more like a pro. The letter is more likely to do what you want it to do. Of course, you should not spend hours or days on every simple letter. But the more important the letter, the more important it is to take time to plan, research, and organize so that the letter will be effective.

Think about job application letters, for example. Suppose you write several letters quickly (without taking time to plan, research, organize, create, edit, and shine before you submit them). You have wasted time and effort if those letters do not result in job interviews. A poorly written cover letter, for example, may mean that the attached résumé may never get opened. Once you have done all the work for one letter, the next ones can almost be copied with only a little time needed to think SMART (e.g., Is this the same type of audience? Are the same skills required?). You may want to create a file of good letters that you can use as models. Many senior managers do this. You can always look online for good examples of well-written letters (e.g., cover letters, letters of resignation, thank you letters).

Keep your letter as short as possible. Business people usually read one-page letters as soon as they open them; they put longer letters (especially those of more than two pages) into the in-basket to read when they have more time (which is almost never!).

MEMOS

Memos are a vital part of a business environment, and if you are working in a hospital or other health care agency, you will likely have to write memos as part of your job. However, traditional memos are disappearing from common use in most health agencies, except, for example, in legal situations. In most agencies, memos may routinely be done by email, but there are still times when a formal printed memo is more appropriate. Formal memos usually deal with more serious matters and nonroutine situations, such as a need to incorporate a new policy or agency recommendation, for example about an outbreak of *Clostridioides difficile* infection. On the other hand, communications between two colleagues confirming a time for lunch are better handled as emails. Thinking SMART will help you.

Memos have "rules," however, and you need to understand the rules of this route. Many rules are similar to those for letters. For formal memos in some agencies, you may need to use all the parts of a business letter, including file numbers. A basic format for a memo is shown in Box 5.4. Essential items in a memo include the following: date; receiver's identity and department; copies (cc) with the receiver's identity and department; sender's identity and departmental address, including telephone number and email address; subject statement; and, most importantly, the message, finishing with recommendations for follow-up. Optional items in a hard-copy memo include the following: signature, copies sent and to whom, enclosures or attachments, stenographic reference, file numbers, and security classification (in agencies where documents must be kept confidential).

BOX 5.4   Sample Memo (hard copy, but this could be an e-memo)

Well Known Hospital
54321 Major Drive
Well Known City, BC V4Z X0O
Telephone (604) 555-0122
Email library@whn.ca

INTERDEPARTMENTAL MEMO

TO: Mary Winters, Unit Manager C4   DATE: 14/12/2019
FROM: Dee Stanos, Staff Library Volunteer   PHONE: (604) 555-0122 (ext.2378)
SUBJECT: Article on Latex Allergies

You spoke to me some time ago about articles on latex allergies, especially resources related to the current situation. I located an excellent review article by Kelly and Sussman (2017) that deals with your question. The full text of this article is available online through the hospital library Academic Search Complete database (you can use the keywords "latex allergies" to find it quickly or use the doi:10.1016/j.jaip.2017.05.029).

Kelly, K. J., & Sussman, G. (2017). Review and feature article: Latex allergy: Where are we now and how did we get there? *The Journal of Allergy and Clinical Immunology: In Practice*, *5*(5),1212-1216. doi:10.1016/j.jaip.2017.05.029

The website of the Asthma and Allergy Foundation of America (2019) has a posting entitled What Are Latex Cross-Reactive Foods? See https://www.aafa.org/latex-allergy

Both resources comment that those who have latex allergies often have coexisting food allergies (e.g., bananas, avocados, chestnuts, celery, and foods sterilized with ethylene oxide).

If you would like further resources, please send me an email and I will do more searching for you next time I am in the hospital.

Point to Note
This library volunteer did not use APA style for the reference but did provide full information.

Keep your memos short and usually keep them to one subject; it is often more efficient for your readers (always consider the audience) if you send two memos when you have two subjects. Doing so may not seem more convenient for you (source), but if the receiver can jot a short note in reply and return it to you immediately, then you will get the action you want more quickly.

Some agencies still use "round-trip memo forms," which allow you to write the original and one or two copies; they are used for specific purposes, such as when you must keep a file related to that memo. This might be required if you are sending a memo seeking action on a drug error or reporting a patient's fall. You keep the bottom copy for your records (e.g., perhaps attached to the patient's chart) and send the top copies. The receiver writes a reply for you at the bottom of the page, keeps the bottom copy for her or his files, and returns the original. These memos are useful when you must send copies to keep others informed.

In some agencies, memos are meant to be posted on a bulletin board or placed in a permanent file so all staff can review them. If the memo is intended to be posted, use a larger font that is easily readable. If it would be more effective to circulate a memo rather than put it on a communication board, you should attach a circulation list. Remember that each of the SMART elements interacts with and influences the others.

If the message to be posted is not suitable for a memo, then it may be more effective to consider a poster. For example, if you are announcing the time and place of the unit's July 1 picnic, perhaps a single page with flag images would be more appropriate than a memo. On the other hand, a poster would not be appropriate for a hospital policy directive that needs to reach all staff.

As you become more senior in your career, your attitude to and use of memos may change. Most front-line staff who attended our writing workshops reported that they resented memos, perhaps because many management memos come across as "Now hear this" directives. Managers tend to write this way because they have a responsibility to communicate, and "Do this" memos seem quick and effective. When you join the management team, however, you can take action to reduce any negative impact that this type of memo has on staff. For example, when you become a manager, you can try to send fewer memos and have more face-to-face meetings with staff. You can set up headline cards (e.g., "New Directives from Pharmacy") and then post all policy memos from Pharmacy in that section of a bulletin board. Or you may choose to file them in a location where staff know to review them. You can read incoming memos yourself and use a highlighter to emphasize relevant points for your staff. These hints, however, relate more to management techniques than to writing skills.

The important point is to think SMART when it comes to writing memos. If you make them short, simple, clear, approachable, appropriate, and easy for the receiver to handle, your memos will be effective.

ELECTRONIC COMMUNICATIONS

Today, many forms of electronic communication allow you to contact others anytime, anywhere, and in many ways. Email messages, instant messaging, social networking, and blogs are some current types of electronic communications.

Email Messages

Within many hospitals and agencies, email messages have replaced telephone calls, informal memos, and business letters. However, email messages are a form of written communication, and the SMART elements apply. Messages to communicate with friends are likely informal, perhaps with contractions and added emoticons. Business messages, including communications with your instructors, need a more formal tone (please reread Chapter 1 on tone because instructors commonly tell us that students are much too informal in their messages). Professional email messages are usually formal, written in professional language, and include any e-memos and e-letters as attachments (rather than in the body of the email). Within agencies, email is used because it is quicker than interdepartmental mail and less intrusive than telephone calls; it also provides a paper trail for future reference. Between agencies, it is often used because it is cheaper than long-distance telephone calls and faster than regular post office delivery or couriers.

Most email messages should be relatively short. If a message is longer than can be read on a single screen, the receiver will have to scroll through it, which is time-consuming, so keep your email message to the point. Remember, email is often read on a mobile device with a tiny screen. Many busy people receive numerous business emails in a day, and they appreciate short, clear, and business-like content. (Consider your audience.)

The format both for sending and receiving email documents is determined by the software programs or telecommunications system that supplies your online service. When the message arrives, most formats are similar to a memo page, with a "From:" line clearly identifying the sender; some recipients do not open messages if they cannot identify the sender. This is followed by a "Date:" line, a "To:" line that gives the receiver's email address, and a "Subject:" line in which you describe briefly what the message will be about. Some systems automatically send all messages without a subject line to a Junk folder or Spam filter. The systems will also do this if the subject line is questionable. The format for sending also allows you to send "Copies" (cc) or "Blind copies" (bcc). Be sure you use these wisely. If you are sending the same email to a group of individuals, you may want to put all the email addresses in the Bcc field; this protects privacy.

Many receivers are concerned about junk mail, confidentiality, security, and privacy. Some receivers delete messages unread if they are sent by a group that does not interest them, or if the subject line indicates something frivolous or unimportant. Be certain you describe the contents appropriately in the subject line if you are sending a message to someone who does not know you by your email address or username. Remember, too, email messages can carry viruses and recipients do not want to take a chance if the sender and subject are not clear.

Many people automatically delete messages once they have dealt with them, and most do not print messages routinely. Be aware your messages may not be kept.

You can also send your message to several receivers all at the same time (through the copy or group-send method); this is a wonderful way to deal with items you want to send to a specific group (e.g., announcements of meetings, agendas, minutes). You can also "Forward" messages to others simply at the click of a button. Remember to limit copies and forwarded mail only to those who need the information, however, or you may gain a reputation as someone who sends junk mail.

Most email programs allow the receiver to "Reply" with a single button. This is another reason why you should keep your message short and limit it to one topic. Be aware of the differences between "Reply" and "Reply All." The latter allows you to send your response to everyone who received the message, including all those who received cc copies; this may not be an appropriate response if you need only reply to the sender—and this will clog up the inboxes of many busy people. Further, using the "Reply All" option when you meant to use "Reply" is often a cause of embarrassment for the sender. (Or worse, some people have been fired when they accidentally used "Reply All" and inappropriate content went to a manager!) Use "Reply All" with caution.

You will no doubt be familiar with the emotional conversational styles (tone) that can be conveyed in an email. For example, use of all CAPITAL LETTERS is generally considered "shouting." You will often see typing errors and common errors (such as *very*) in informal email messages. Depending on your audience and how formal your message needs to be, you should probably proofread before you press "Send."

You can also send business letters by email, especially when you are eager to have the message arrive quickly. You can do this by attaching a file containing the letter. Or if it is a short letter, you can place it in the body of the email. In such cases, after you have filled in the opening boxes, you should format the message exactly as you would a business letter. You can even use a simple letterhead with your name, address, telephone number, and email address at the top of the page, the date and inside address, and then a line that says "Letter sent by email" just above the salutation.

If you are sending the letter as an attachment, you should probably save it in your computer, giving it a clear, descriptive file name. You would then send the file attached to a brief email message, saying something like "Letter attached as file named < gzletter.doc >"; this alerts the receiver to the fact that there is a named file attached so that he or she can easily retrieve it later from the document files in the computer. If the letter is vital, you may want to send a hard copy as backup.

You should know how to set up a "digital signature line" so receivers will have your contact information easily available (plus you will save time typing this information as it will load automatically). You need not include an electronic signature (unless it is legally required, as for scholarships, bursaries, and grant applications).

Use the SMART principles. Is the email route suitable for your message? Do you need to transfer printed information quickly? Does the format matter? The basic email format is best suited for short messages, and you can attach files or documents. For example, you can send an assignment or a report via email as an attached file, which can then be printed by the receiver if desired or required. This method works wonderfully for the exchange of draft documents, but often the formatting is not suitable for finished documents. You also need to consider whether your receiver likes to use email and file transfer.

Instant Messaging

Another form of two-way electronic communication is instant messaging (e.g., texting, online chat, Skype, Google Docs) that allows real-time discussion or exchange over the Internet. Instant messages are more immediate and direct than email, making them seem more like speech. Text, video, images, and audio can all be shared through instant messaging, usually using apps (e.g., WhatsApp, Facebook Messenger).

Many instant messages are written text, so you need good writing skills for clear communication. Because they are commonly used for short, informal exchanges between friends (source and audience), a more congenial tone is usually acceptable. The use of acronyms (usually written in all capital letters), emoticons, and abbreviations, which often convey a personable tone, is more common in instant messaging than in other forms of written communication. If you choose to use acronyms, know the language and avoid the trap of trying to sound more up-to-date than you are. Acronyms often change overnight and you will look foolish if you riddle your text with outdated slang or shorthand. If in doubt, consult a current website of common acronyms (or ask your teenager). Currently, LOL (laughing out loud), ROFL (rolling on the floor laughing), NP (no problem), and IMHO (in my humble opinion) seem to be up-to-date; by the time you read this they may be passé.

Sarcasm and attempts at humour can be misinterpreted in words on a screen, so avoid these unless you know the person receiving your text (audience) well. Even though the dialogue is brief, it is still courteous to begin and end your instant message with a short salutation and sign-off. A sign-off makes it clear that from your perspective the message exchange is completed. Being courteous also means waiting for a response to your comment before continuing. If you send a second message before receiving a response to your first message, it becomes confusing and you will be unsure to which message the receiver is responding. Attend to grammar, punctuation, and spelling since all writing, even instant messaging, reflects on you. Sloppy writing can be interpreted as not caring about, or disrespecting, the receiver (audience). But often in informal messaging, you do not need to waste time and energy editing if you are just asking someone if he or she is ready to go for lunch.

Social Networking

Do you use social media sites such as Twitter, Facebook, LinkedIn, or Instagram to communicate with others? Social networking has become a ubiquitous form of electronic communication that uses Internet-based programs to facilitate professional and personal connections. It now has a role within professional courses, sometimes as a teaching or learning strategy or even as part of an assignment using modern skills to communicate with patients or colleagues. Social networks allow you to share messages with large numbers of people (including people you do not know) at one time. Social media has also become a common channel for marketing and fundraising. Successful social networking depends in part on excellent writing skills. For example, creating a tweet on your Twitter account that will be read and retweeted, or getting a "like," "share," or positive comment on your Facebook post, involves more than just typing a set number of characters. You must consider the source element as you compose your message if you want to reach a large audience and achieve maximum exposure for your ideas (and a favourable response).

Each social networking channel (route) has rules about what you can send (e.g., size of image, number of characters, appropriate content). You should craft your message to suit the platform you are using. For example, you can use hashtags— short links beginning with a hash, also called a pound or number sign (#)—which turn keywords into searchable terms within Twitter or Instagram posts. If you want to tell a longer story Facebook is a more suitable platform. Generally, if you want to engage your potential audience (using any social media route), include catchy titles or headings and ensure your well-written messages are original, timely, and newsworthy.

Skillfully crafting your message for the platform you choose will increase the probability your ideas will be read and shared widely. Beginning with a question or quotation can be one way to get a potential reader's attention and increase your "likes," "shares," or "clicks" and maybe even affect your mark. Shorter messages are more often read. Tweets are short because of character limits but you can potentially write many words in Facebook; however, shorter Facebook messages are preferred by your potential audience (social media researchers suggest 40 characters or less is optimum). Keep in mind that Instagram captions have a size limit of 2200 characters, but only the first three lines of text appear before the remainder of your message is hidden. Again, shorter posts will be more appealing to a target audience. Including an appropriate, appealing image and staying positive are also strategies to get your posts noticed and shared. Finally, hashtags help people find and follow you on social media. They help organize content that is continuously changing, and they provide a means to track discussions on a specific topic; learning to create effective hashtags is a mini-course in itself.

Blogs

A blog is an ongoing series of entries on a website, often devoted to a specific topic, that is regularly updated by an author or small group. A blog is usually created for a specific audience and is written in a conversational tone. Posts within a blog appear in reverse chronological order, with the most recent content appearing at the top. Blogs may include a space where readers can add comments. If you are interested in starting a blog, WordPress.com and Blogger.com are examples of free services that can help you get started. Blogs are used as assignments in some courses. You might be asked to use the blog format to share your original ideas on a course topic and then to share your blog with the class so that others can read and comment on your work. You could also be asked to collaborate with a group of other students to create a blog that might be used for teaching patients or colleagues about a topic. Such blogs could include scholarly content embellished with images and other graphics. These may be assigned as an alternative to a traditional essay or report. Instructors use these types of assignments to increase your digital fluency.

With blogs, as with all types of electronic communication, the SMART elements will guide you to success. For example, before you begin to blog, consider your target audience. If you know about your audience (especially what will interest them), you will have a good start when deciding what your message should be.

Craft your message so it will be appealing and begin with an engaging and informative title. The title needs to give your potential audience sufficient information so they know if it is worth reading further. Once you hook readers with your title, make the first few lines of your blog post compelling. Tell a story, include an image, share a humorous incident, or begin with an intriguing or surprising fact. Too much content or poorly organized material overwhelms, tires, and bores readers. Appropriate use of lists or point-form breaks content into manageable segments. Remember successful blogs have new content added often, but the content needs to be worth reading. A well-designed blog post looks different (and has a much different tone) than does a scholarly essay! Finally, edit your posts before you share them. The PROCESS steps described in Chapter 2 apply equally to blog posts.

CLASS PRESENTATIONS

Frequently in your courses, especially in more advanced courses, you, perhaps with one or two classmates, may be asked to "present" a paper. Although, strictly speaking, a class presentation is not a written communication but an oral communication, you will find it helpful to use the SMART elements (Chapter 1) and to follow the PROCESS steps (Chapter 2). If you use computer-created visuals (e.g., PowerPoint, Prezi, Keynote) to accompany your presentation, then it is essential that you consider the SMART elements and PROCESS steps. It is surprising how gigantic a spelling error or incorrect punctuation mark looks when it is projected onto the big screen! Careful writing, followed by thorough editing, is the best way to prevent this demoralizing situation.

For most students, a good oral presentation starts with written notes. You may even want to write out a full copy of what you wish to say; perhaps you even will be required to hand this in to your instructor. Usually, what you need, however, is a precise and detailed written outline.

As always, you need to pay special attention to your audience and route. In an oral presentation, route includes awareness of the venue in which you will be presenting. For example, the audience may be a few classmates, some agency staff members, or maybe a small group of patients in a hospital cafeteria, or it may be a large assembly in an auditorium in which you need a microphone, a podium, and audiovisual aids. Time is an essential part of the route in an oral presentation, just as length is an important part of a written presentation. You usually will have been allotted a specific time (e.g., 15 minutes with 5 minutes for questions). You must stick with this. Keep this timing in mind even as you begin the writing PROCESS. Tone is also an important consideration. The wording in oral presentations usually is less formal than in written presentations, but there is a difference between chatty presentations full of slang and structured, lecture-like presentations. The vocabulary you use must be appropriate to the audience; for example, if you are giving a presentation about diabetes to a group of multicultural patients, consider that English may be a second language.

You still follow the PROCESS, but after the Outline step you can become more creative with the message you want to cover (or, if it is a specific assigned topic, that you are required to cover). What you do is create a series of speaker's notes, usually in point form and in a large font so that you can refer to them easily during the presentation if you get anxious. From these notes, you will make your presentation without "reading it aloud"; reading from a paper is dreadfully boring for your audience unless you are an excellent actor.

In the Create step and the Editing step, develop a series of specific major points that you plan to cover; in an oral presentation, these can be presented as "point form." Although you would not use point form in most written papers, it can be meaningful and valuable in oral presentations. You also need to develop some phrases or sentences that will make an impression on your audience. You may wish to highlight these in your notes so they will stand out easily as you do your presentation. In the Shine step, rehearse your oral presentation aloud; you probably will want to do this several times, and, if possible, practise on an audience of a few trustworthy friends or family members. They can give you feedback but ask them to do this tactfully at the end of the trial presentation. You could practise in front of a mirror, or video yourself practising and watch it, if you cannot get an audience.

Just as with a written presentation (see Chapter 2), you will have an introduction (during which you clearly state what you are going to tell them so they understand the purpose and aim of your presentation). Then you will have the main body of your message, with as many details or points as you need and have time for; these are, once again, divided into logical, well-organized sections. And you will conclude with a brief, but beautifully worded, summary during which you reiterate what you told them.

As you research your topic and prepare your notes, do not neglect to prepare citations and references for any primary sources that you use. Most probably, your instructor will want you to hand in a reference list or bibliography. You may even want to prepare "handouts" (photocopies) for the audience. Including references in handouts is a good idea or you can list them on a final slide.

Depending on the message and the route, you may wish to use visual aids. For example, if it is an intimate presentation for new mothers on a labour and delivery unit, you may want to use a whiteboard, hang up a poster board, hand out educational materials, or use a doll as a demonstration baby. For presentations to larger groups, you may wish to use a computer-based presentation complete with images, text slides, websites, and video or audio clips. More than 40 different computer software programs for creating presentations are available, each with different features; some have associated costs. If you decide to create a presentation, do some research and find the program that suits your message and audience. Examples of programs available include Zoho Show, Visme, Haiku Deck, Emaze, Keynote, Projeqt, Slidebean, Slide Dog, Prezi, and PowerPoint.

Computer-generated presentations have many of the same qualities as other special written communications, with their own rules of the route. Start with a title slide. Use a font size large enough so your text can be read easily from all parts of the room. Prepare some of your "points" in text using the computer software, which will help you set up "bullets" or other typographical devices. You also can incorporate illustrations, photographs, audio clips, video clips, or webpages. Be sure you balance graphics and text and use a pleasing contrast between the background colour and the text; avoid using a busy ("noisy") background. Consider the length of time for your presentation and use an appropriate number of visual materials.

Just as with any other route, you can find whole books on how to do different types of oral presentations, ranging from brief toasts, to informative talks, to formal speeches. We have found, however, that excellent information is available on the Internet. We googled "how to do class presentations," and found helpful guidelines on university sites (e.g., University of Kent [UK], University of Hawaii, and Mount Royal University).

As you get ready to take the Submit step of the PROCESS ladder, be sure that you check out the room and equipment you will be using; do this well in advance of the time for your presentation. You do not want to arrive with your presentation saved on a flash drive only to find you should have submitted it earlier to a technician as an attached file. If you can, do your presentation without a microphone or lapel mic, it usually is better to avoid using one. However, if you are soft-spoken and the room is large, then you must use a microphone. If you use a stationary mic, you should not wander during your presentation.

A final point: Once you are ready to present, take a deep breath, look around at your audience, and make eye contact—and then give everyone your biggest smile. All that will relax you, and you will be better prepared to give a great presentation.

RÉSUMÉS AND CURRICULUM VITAE

Two important written communications you will need during your career are a résumé and a curriculum vitae (Latin term for *course of life*). A résumé (sometimes the word is written without the accents) is a brief summary of educational and employment experiences that is submitted with a job application. In today's world, chances are that you will change jobs during your working lifetime *at least* six times; many health care professionals hold up to 15 different jobs during their careers. Sometimes these changes are within a single agency, but sometimes you may even decide to change to a different field. A curriculum vitae (CV) is longer than a résumé and is a comprehensive record of all your education, jobs, qualifications (professional licensure and relevant memberships), publications, grants, presentations, and honours. The differences between the two relate to purpose, length, layout, and information supplied.

A résumé is so important for that first job after graduation that your instructor often gives you an assignment on preparing a résumé, and it will become more and more important in later years. Hospitals and most other health care agencies also require you to fill out an application form designed for the institution; the form makes it easy for a personnel officer to review information quickly and assess your qualifications for the job. If that is the case, you must fill out the form, but you can also attach your résumé, which carries additional weight and shows that you know something about job hunting. Furthermore, if you have your résumé on hand when you fill out the application form, you are more likely to have all the necessary information (e.g., dates). So you should develop a résumé, or at least a worksheet that you can follow when filling out applications, soon after graduation. This initial résumé will eventually grow into a basic CV. Templates for résumés are available online or you can hire people to help you prepare a résumé, but if you learn how to do it yourself, by thinking SMART, you may end up with a much better message.

To develop a good résumé and keep it up to date so that you can apply for positions in coming years, consider starting a professional portfolio, either in hard copy or online (an e-portfolio). The portfolio not only contains your résumé or job history but also a collection of documents (sometimes called "artefacts" or, in the United States, "artifacts") that demonstrate your abilities for a potential employer. Initially, you can include all important background materials you will need in future years, such as a high school certificate, graduation certificates, registration examination results, copies of official documents pertaining to courses and marks, and information on special courses taken (e.g., CPR certificate). These documents will come in handy for many years and will help you to keep dates correct. (Believe us, you will forget such information!) Later, it may include such items as your photograph (usually a head-and-shoulders photo) and copies of pamphlets, reports, work-relevant presentations, papers, or videos you may have prepared during your career. Even if you do not submit a portfolio to the employer when you first apply for a position, you can take it with you to your job interview or add a link to your e-portfolio on your résumé.

A résumé is usually your first contact with a potential employer, so you need to consider your audience. Most employers spend less than a minute looking over a résumé when it first arrives, so consider how to make yours stand out in a pile of other résumés. You could print it in fancy type on shocking pink paper with a colour copy of your photo at the top, or use a geometric background on your electronic résumé, but does such a résumé convey the nonverbal message you want to send? Such a résumé might be useful if you are applying to an advertising agency or talent bureau, but most health care employers expect a more professional approach. For most health care employers, your résumé should be short, clear, well organized, and neat so that the essential points can be assessed quickly.

You need to consider some important things about yourself as a source. If you are looking during a tight job market, you may need to send out several résumés at once. If your budget is slim, and the employer asked for a printed copy, you may wish to develop a general résumé that can be used for several potential employers, such as several hospitals in an urban area. Often employers will ask for an electronic résumé submitted with an online job application form. If so, you may wish to develop a good general format but adapt each résumé to fit the needs of each potential employer, such as a pediatric unit, a home care agency, or a geriatric facility.

If you do not deliver your résumé in person or attach it to a job application, you may attach a brief covering letter. Its main message simply says, using the appropriate words, that you are enclosing (or attaching) a résumé for consideration; if you are applying for a specific job, you can add information such as "I would like to apply for the position in your operating room that was recently advertised on the Indeed job site." However, the covering letter also allows you to send the résumé to a particular person, which is always better than addressing a general department (see the section in this chapter on business letters). The covering letter also allows you to provide a bit of additional personal information and to indicate that you would like to have a job interview. You can add such information as the best ways to reach you (by telephone or email). This kind of information is not suitable in the résumé itself.

A résumé alone will not get you a job. The purpose of a résumé is to get you a job interview. Potential employers develop a short list of candidates based on their résumés (or application forms), so you should know how to develop a good one and supply all the important information in one or two pages.

Content for Résumés and CVs

Most résumés fall into one of two broad categories: chronological and functional. The chronological résumé is the most common and concentrates on supplying all of the more basic details about your education and employment history. The functional résumé allows you to include more about various jobs you have held. Infographic résumés, which include images and other design elements to supplement written text, are becoming more common; colour, format, icons, pictures, and various fonts are used to convey content in a short and more pictorial form. Professional health employers tend to prefer traditional types of résumés.

You need to keep information suitable for both types in your résumé file or your professional portfolio because this material will be useful when you fill out applications and when you go to interviews. However, the basic content is similar for both and includes the following categories: (1) name and contact information, (2) education, (3) work experience, (4) honours, (5) professional memberships, (6) publications, (7) personal information, (8) references and contact information, and (9) dates. Sample résumés are shown in Boxes 5.5 and 5.6.

BOX 5.5   Sample Chronological Résumé (New Graduate)

NOEL KANE, R.N.
Apt. 12 — 1812 Bayview Street
Surrey, BC V4B 0X0
Telephone: (604) 555-0144 (home), (604) 555-0172 (cell)
Email: reachnoel@cattle.net

Job Objective:	Registered Nurse Staff Position, Surrey District Hospital	
Education:		
	2019	Registered Nurse Degree
		School of Nursing
		Chinook Community College
		Sardis, BC
	2015	High School Graduation (with honors)
		Duke of Connaught Senior Secondary
		South Surrey, BC
Work Background:		
	2018	(Feb.)–2019 (June) Kitchen Assistant (weekend relief)
		Sardis Memorial Hospital, Sardis, BC
	2017	(June–July) Kitchen Assistant
		Sardis Memorial Hospital, Sardis, BC
Awards:		
	2016	University Women's Club (South Fraser Branch)
		Ethel Singh Scholarship ($1,000 for further study)
Professional Memberships:		
	2019	College of Registered Nurses of BC
	2015–2019	Canadian Student Nurses Association
		(national vice-president, 2018–19)
References:		
Mr. J. R. Toews	R.R.3, Box 17, Sardis, BC V6M 0X1	
	(604) 555-0152	
	toews@zmail.com	
Mrs. Cheryl Jones	School of Nursing, Chinook Community College,	
	Sardis, BC V7K 1X0	
	(604) 555-0181, local 546	
	jonesch@CCC.edu	

(Prepared August 2019)

Point to Note
Noel Kane chose to use periods in R.N., a style decision, but see also Box 5.6.

BOX 5.6   Sample Functional Résumé (Recent Graduate)

MARTHA CHUNG, RN, BSN
Apt. 91 — 2488 Johnston Road
Edmonton, AB T6G 0X0
Telephone: (403) 555-0136 (home), (870) 555-0131 (cell)

Job Objective: Unit Manager, Post-Anaesthetic Recovery Unit, Edmonton General

Work Background:

2019	(June)–present	RN staff duties in 18-bed PAR
	Staff Nurse	Responsible for orientation of new staff
	PAR Unit	
	Edmonton General	Developed CPR Cart for Emergency Unit and for Main Building
2015	(Aug.)–2019 (May)	RN staff duties in a 24-bed, 24-hour
	Staff Nurse	Emergency Unit
	Emergency Department	During last six months worked permanent
	Queenston General	night duty (1900–0700 hours) and was senior
	Queenston, ON	nurse-in-charge

Education:

2015 (June)	CPR Certification Course, Boston University Hospital, Boston (five-week specialty course)
2015	Bachelor of Science in Nursing (with honours) Faculty of Nursing King's University Queenston, ON

Professional Memberships:

College and Association of Registered Nurses of Alberta

College of Nurses of Ontario

Publications:

Chow, E. K., & Chung, M. (2018). Safety precautions for crash cart medications. *RN Communiqué, 4*(3), 6–7.

Personal Information:

Age 28 years, married with one child
Fluent in Cantonese
Hobbies: five-pin bowling, swimming (Red Cross Life-Saving Certificate)

References:

Available on request

(Prepared August 2019)

You can also develop a combination résumé, which contains elements of both the chronological and functional categories. For more information and some examples, you can refer to the University of Toronto Mississauga website or the Harvard University website (both are listed in the References at the end of this chapter).

NAME AND CONTACT INFORMATION

These should be given clearly at the top of the first page. You are not required and do not usually supply personal information (e.g., marital status, family, age, weight, height, etc.) in the résumé and never at the top, but this is a judgement you make as the source. Note that in Box 5.6, Martha Chung decided to include personal information; she probably would not have done so if she were sending this to a large hospital, other than to highlight her language skills.

EDUCATION

List the highlights of your education in reverse chronological order. When you graduate and are applying for your first positions, you may want to include your high school graduation, although employers will know college or university graduates will have completed high school. As you determine whether to include high school graduation, think SMART: source (are you young, inexperienced, and applying for a first position, or are you older, experienced, and applying for a senior position?); message (is your educational experience or your work experience more important to this potential employer?); audience (would this information be relevant to this reader?); route (have you room to include all the details?); and tone (is this a *formal* application in which you should include all relevant information?).

Information about relevant noncredit education may also be included in this section, such as information about short courses (e.g., CPR, advanced life support, neonatal care). You definitely would include information on certifications and specialty courses.

WORK EXPERIENCE

This section of your résumé will change most throughout your career. At first, you will not have much to include, but you should regularly update your files and CV, even if you do not need a new résumé for each new job.

If you are at an early stage in your career, you may wish to include information on part-time work, even if it does not seem relevant to the job for which you are applying. One personnel officer advised us that when he is reviewing for entry-level positions, he notes whether the applicant had worked summers at fast-food outlets such as McDonald's or A&W; he said that applicants who have held those jobs probably have a good overall work ethic. If your high school or your faculty arranged co-op placements, practicums, or internships, you may want to give details about these. Volunteer work should be mentioned in this section as well; for example, if you worked every Thursday after classes throughout high school as a volunteer on a unit of the hospital to which you are applying, you should include this information.

When you are further along in your career, you would list your various positions in reverse chronological order. You could separate positions to mark advancements, even though these positions were for the same employer. For example:

2017–present	Manager of Rehabilitation Therapy, Peace Arch Hospital, White Rock
2015–2017	Physiotherapist, Peace Arch Hospital, White Rock

Later in your career, when you need to list several positions, you would combine these two and probably would combine these on your CV as it gets longer.

HONOURS

In this section, which should be brief and to the point, you can include scholarships and awards.

PROFESSIONAL MEMBERSHIPS

You need to include information about your professional registration and indicate jurisdictions where you are licensed. If you are hired, you will need to provide your professional registration or licensure number, but this important and confidential information should not appear on the résumé. In some professions, your provincial or state registration implies membership in your national association, you can decide whether to mention this membership or not. You should include current professional memberships, and you may elect to include some or all past professional memberships. For example, if you held office in a professional association in another province or state, but are no longer a member, this information may still be relevant because it indicates involvement in professional activities. You would not usually include membership in community service organizations or social groups, religious organizations, or sports activities, unless you believe that they are relevant to your audience and your message. You would include these on your CV as your career progresses.

PUBLICATIONS

In this section, you list professional publications. Early in your career, you may not have many. If you eventually go into academia, the list of publications on your CV will be long. You should not trim this section; that list of publications should be complete and uncensored, even if an article eventually seems immature or unimportant. In later years, you may wish to put a lengthy publication list on separate sheets and attach it to your résumé only when relevant.

PERSONAL INFORMATION

This section creates controversy. You are not required to give information such as age, marital status, or number of children, but sometimes this information is relevant (see Box 5.6). For example, if you are seeking a daytime job because you have a child and wish to be home in the evenings, you may want to make this point on your résumé (and in your covering letter). Many people believe that information about hobbies should never be included, but if you and your potential employer share a mutual hobby or interest it might make that person take a more careful (or positive) look at your submission. Information about extracurricular activities gives a potential employer an idea of the person behind the facts. Obviously, you have to think SMART and make up your own mind.

REFERENCES AND CONTACT INFORMATION

Inclusion of references with a résumé is another controversial point. Some agencies require that you supply them; others prefer to get in touch with one or more of your previous employers directly. It is certainly appropriate to write "References available on request," or you can simply omit this section. If you do use names, you should first ask these individuals if they are willing to give you positive recommendations. If you do not list reference contacts on your résumé, bring a paper with names and contact information (including email addresses) to the interview. If you are asked for a list of references, you will look well prepared when you hand your list to the interviewer.

DATE

Résumés and CVs should be dated, usually at the bottom of the last page, to show they are current. You need not sign résumés or CVs.

Helpful Hints About Résumés and CVs

- Be accurate and truthful. Prospective employers may check the information. Furthermore, your résumé or CV may form part of your permanent work record. Do not exaggerate or try to oversell yourself.
- Be as brief as possible in a résumé. One page is good; two full pages are maximum (even for senior administrators). Applicants for teaching positions at universities may use longer résumés or offer a CV.
- Double-check grammar, spelling, and punctuation. Use action words (e.g., developed, coordinated, supervised) when possible. Use point form or use short paragraphs and keep the same verb tense throughout.
- Pay attention to visual presentation. A résumé should never look cramped—and should never be soiled or messy.
- Use a covering letter.
- Do not underestimate yourself. A résumé is an advertisement for you; it is intended to get you an interview.

REPORTS

A business report is another standard route of communication for health professionals. Reports require the same SMART thinking and follow the same PROCESS as other written communications. The report is used when the message is longer and requires more detailed background than would be given in a memo or letter. The tone tends to be more formal, although a report can range from slightly informal (between two departments working on a project) to highly formal (royal commission or congressional report to a federal government; brief to a provincial or state government). The audience can vary from a single individual to the general public. Reports tend to be shared with larger groups, so there is a primary audience (the person or small group for whom the report was created) and a secondary audience (the larger group with whom the primary audience may share the report). An annual report from a unit manager to the vice-president of patient care may end up being shared with the executive committee, the financial department, and the president of the hospital auxiliary and may even be reproduced in the hospital's annual report to the public. Hence, a good starting point for a person asked to prepare a report is to find out exactly who needs the report (primary and secondary audiences) and what its purpose is to be.

In other words, if you are asked to prepare a report, you need to follow the writing PROCESS, especially the first three steps. As part of your research, get copies of previous reports that may help you to understand the particular format used in your agency, but get other kinds of reports as well so that you can make innovative and creative changes. Obviously, if you are a hospital unit manager preparing a quarterly report, you will keep it simpler in format and layout than if you are preparing a report about a disciplinary action for a professional association.

Remember, however, that the message is the point of a written communication. Be certain that you understand the message and its purpose. Are you asked to provide a report with data on various brands of infant cots so that a committee of several managers can decide? Or are you asked to recommend the brand of infant cots that should be purchased based on your research and expertise? In the former, you will need to provide all the background details on various infant cots available, including costs, safety factors, ease of use, and other such details, so the committee can debate the issue and make an informed decision; the purpose of this report is to save the committee time. In the latter, you can be more direct and state that, based on your research and testing and after consideration of prices, you (an expert source) recommend the "Babe Cot" as the most suitable of six cots currently on the market. You might choose to support your recommendation briefly in the report and to include appendices that give background information on all the cots, but the main body of the report should be brief, to the point, and based on your expertise because the purpose of your report is to recommend. In the latter instance, the committee might simply approve your report and forward it to the purchasing department, so you should include the details the matériels manager will need to make the order.

For reports in which you are asked to give an opinion or recommendation, you can use the acronym PRESS:

Position: state your position clearly.
Reason: state the reason you are for or against.

Example: give an example or two to illustrate your position.
Support: reinforce your position with statistics and facts.
Summarize: close with a brief statement of your position.

Some reports fall halfway between the informational report and the recommendation report; these are termed "interpretive reports," which not only inform and describe but also analyze. The interpretive report, however, does not usually make recommendations. Progress reports fall into this category.

Proposals, including grant proposals and project requests, are also kinds of reports. Important sections of these include proposed costs (budget) and methods of implementation; a time schedule is also useful. If you are applying for a grant, a foundation usually requires you to fill out specific forms; check before starting work (i.e., during the Plan step of PROCESS). As part of planning, you may also want to borrow (or, if report writing is going to be a major part of your job, even buy) a book, or find a reputable web resource, on how to write reports. Yes, there are books and websites on how to write reports and even on how to write certain kinds of reports (e.g., proposals, technical reports). This section provides only an overview.

Format of a Report

A good report follows the traditional outline—introduction, body, conclusion—with one slight difference. In most written communications, the introduction merely "tells them what you are going to tell them" in broad terms. In a report, the introduction *summarizes* what you are going to tell your audience and is specific about conclusions, recommendations, and actions to be taken. In other words, you give the essence of the report on the first page.

You provide a summary at the beginning because of the audience. For many readers of a business report, the summary is all that is required. If the reader needs more details, he or she can go deeper into the report, but most readers do not want to read the whole report to discover "the bottom line." Furthermore, the report is organized to make it easy, through presentation, for a reader to find needed details.

If you share a link to your report during a meeting, and the chair allows members time to look at the report, observe how they react. Typically, about 80% of committee members will turn quickly to page 1 and begin to read. If the opening on page 1 catches their interest, they will continue to read all of page 1 and go on to page 2. About 40% of typical committee members continue to read page 2 (provided the message stays relevant); the other 60% will let their attention wander, flip or scroll through the rest of the report (many will go to the end to look for conclusions), or turn to other committee matters. Only about 10% will continue to read on to page 3. The same pattern is followed when people get your report in their offices; about 80% of them turn immediately to page 1. They will stay with it for page 2 and maybe page 3 and then set the report aside to read when they have more time (which, for most busy people, is never). Thus, where should you put the important message in your report?

In the past, reports typically began with all the background, went through the history of why the report was needed, and built up to the conclusion on the last few pages. Today, reports start with conclusions and recommendations, followed by the reasons for the recommendations, and the background and historical perspective (if included at all) tend to be near the end. The former style is still used in some contexts, usually for expository or traditional reports; the latter style is considered motivational and is more likely to be used in hospitals and health care agencies.

The standard organization for a detailed report would thus follow this route (you will probably notice similarities to student assignments):

- **cover** (if necessary), with a good, catchy title
- **title page(s)**, including information on authors or compilers, place, date, and other relevant material (e.g., contact information)
- **preliminary pages**, including, if the report is more than 20 pages, a table of contents (and perhaps also a list of tables, graphs, or illustrations); in major reports, you may also need a preface and acknowledgements (but keep them brief)
- **introduction**—frequently titled "Executive Summary"—in which the report is summarized in one or, at most, two pages; this summary may even be put before the preliminary pages to make it stand out
- **body of the report**, which includes some or all these elements:
  - synopsis or abstract of the body
  - background (the *why* of this report)
  - method used to look into the subject (how you did it)
  - findings (with all the facts, including financial information)
  - discussion (including interpretation of facts, recommendations in detail, and conclusions in detail)
  - concluding section of the body (which ties the whole report together and reiterates the executive summary)

- **references and bibliography**
- **appendices** (these come *after* references and bibliography if you did not create them)

Not all reports will follow this format, of course; it depends on Source * Message * Audience * Route * Tone. For example, some hospital administrations require quarterly and annual reports from department heads and have strict rules about format. One hospital vice-president asked department heads to organize their quarterly reports this way:

1. Brief introductory statement followed by sections on progress since the last report (were goals met?)

2. Body, giving statements and comparison figures on:
   2.1 budget
   2.2 staffing
   2.3 administrative problems
   2.4 in-service education activities
   2.5 committee participation
   2.6 other relevant activities

3. Concluding section with a list of new long- and short-term goals.

This vice-president also wanted department heads to use a modified Harvard numbering style whereby each section in the body of the report used her specific numbering system and each paragraph in each section had a number. Thus, the first paragraph in the budget section was 2.1.1, the second paragraph was numbered 2.1.2, and so on. The department heads knew exactly what was expected by this particular audience and could prepare their reports accordingly.

Short Reports ("Briefs")

The noun "brief" came into business use during the 1990s. Generally speaking, a brief is a short report usually recommending some kind of action or solution to a problem. The term has been around much longer in the legal profession, in which a brief is a concise statement intended to inform other, usually more senior, counsellors about a client's case. No doubt you have also heard the term used in military and government circles in the form "briefing." The idea is to get a summary of a lot of information into a short, usable form for someone who knows less about a subject than you do but who is in a position to take action.

Professional associations often present briefs to political committees or commissions. A written brief or short report is taken to the committee's meeting, and a representative of the association gives an even briefer oral presentation and answers questions (e.g., to a commission on health care costs). In these instances, a brief is a longer and more formal document than a letter or memo; a brief might contain 750 to 1000 words (three to five pages), which would be a l-o-n-g letter!

The shortest reports can be sent as memos. For example, if a senior administrator in your hospital asks you for a report on the status of a grant given to your department by the hospital auxiliary, he or she probably does not want a formal layout. An example of a short progress report sent as a memo is given in Box 5.7.

BOX 5.7   Sample Short Progress Report (Memo Format)

Well Known Hospital
54321 Major Drive
Well Known City, BC V4Z X0O
Telephone (604) 555-0177
Email doeja@wkh.org

TO: Jane Doe, Vice-President Patient Services
FROM: John Singh, RN, Unit Manager OR   **PHONE:** ext. 123
DATE: 16 March 2019

RE: Progress Report on WKH Auxiliary Special Funding

The Operating Room received a one-time special grant of $13,000 from the WKH Auxiliary in December 2018 to purchase operating room instruments. The purchase is progressing on time and on budget, with instruments worth $11,769 (including relevant taxes, delivery, and so on) ordered and received. When one more back order is received, the rest of the money will have been used.

Background

At a meeting of WKH OR staff, a list was drawn up of instruments often requested by surgeons but frequently unavailable or in short supply. These instruments were in addition to those requested in the 2017–2018 OR budget; some items that had to be cut from the budget were included in this list.

OR staff then prepared a proposal for funding, in consultation with the Matériels Manager. The proposal was supported by the WKH Medical Committee and approved by WKH Administration.

Continued

BOX 5.7 Sample Short Progress Report (Memo Format)—Cont'd

The funding proposal was submitted to the WKH Auxiliary in November, and the Auxiliary approved the $13,000 request at its meeting in early December.
The list included

- special instruments for work in ear surgery now that this specialty is available at WKH; and
- additional basic instruments to help shorten turn-around times for operations.

Orders to Date

On 13 January 2019, three magnifying lenses and a complete set of auricular instruments, including pinna scrapers, antihelix retractors, ossicle retrievers, and tympani forceps, were ordered from Ear-Ache Instruments of New York. These instruments arrived 12 February 2019. One of the magnifying lenses was scratched on arrival and has been returned; a replacement is on its way. All other instruments were checked and incorporated into OR stocks. Total cost of these instruments was $10,343.

A list of 12 special retractors often requested by surgeons was drawn up by OR staff and checked with the Chief of Surgery. The order was placed 19 January 2019 with Retractor-Magic of Montreal and received 19 February. Total cost was $1,426.

An OR micro-sterilizer for auricular instruments has been ordered through 3X Instruments of Germany (there is no North American supplier). The list price is $987 (converted from Euros); this should use most of the remaining funds but remain within the budget. Expected date of delivery is 20 March 2019. Final cost will depend on the exchange rate when the order is received. If the cost exceeds the $13,000 grant, the few extra dollars will be taken from the general OR budget for supplies.

Copies of purchase orders for all items, with prices, are attached for information.

Future Actions

All equipment should be received and in use by 5 April 2019. Once all equipment is received and put into use, letters from the OR Head Nurse, the Chief of Surgery, and the new ENT Specialist will be written and sent to the WKH Auxiliary President outlining the use and thanking members for the grant.

Copy: J. Hancock, Matériels Manager

Helpful Hints About Reports

- Keep your report as short as possible—the briefer the better.
- Summarize your message on page 1.
- Be as brief as possible; use tables to summarize and present information visually; put background details into appendices.
- Keep the purpose of the report in mind—is it to inform, persuade, request, analyze, or recommend?
- Do you want the receivers of the report to take action? If so, be specific about the action you want them to take and request it on page 1.
- Recommend solutions if you identify problems.
- Provide full information related to cost, if relevant; in today's world, report readers are concerned about budgets.

MINUTES AND AGENDAS

At some point in your career, even as a student, you are likely going to be asked to "do" minutes of a meeting—and good luck, especially if you are asked to do this at the last moment without any warning! Minutes are, in essence, one kind of report; they report on what happened during a meeting, and they generally reflect the action taken by the group (what was done rather than what was said). Names of people who move motions are generally required, and the group may want or need to include the names of seconders. Some groups record only whether a motion passed or failed; others wish to have the numbers of people who voted for, against, or abstain; still other groups record all names and how they voted. The tone will vary from highly formal to informal, depending on the group, but generally should sound professional and business-like.

Unfortunately, the rules of the route for minutes are almost as varied as meetings themselves. Minutes vary from sketchy communiqués that give only motions and state passed or defeated to full transcripts, such as the Canadian Parliament's *Hansard* (Parliament of Canada, n.d.) and the U.S. *Congressional Record* (Library of Congress, 2018) that are long, complex records done by trained staff. Other minutes provide a summary of the discussion that occurred on each motion and a summary of committee reports. Still other types of minutes include complete copies of all reports by officers, committee chairs, and other speakers (supplied by these individuals). Such large agencies use *Robert's Rules of Order* (Robert, Robert, Evans, Honemann, & Balch, 2013), which was originally written in 1876 to set rules for military and political meetings and has been in constant use since. *Robert's Rules* is now the most widely used guide for recording minutes of organizations, associations, clubs, and groups throughout North America. An 11th edition was published in 2013, and updated online versions are widely available; these deal with the many changes that have evolved in recent years to deal with online communication and "electronic meetings."

The best advice in a situation where you are asked, without warning, to take minutes is to discuss the style briefly with the chair and determine if there is a preferred template. Then take as complete a set of notes as possible and, later, obtain copies of minutes of previous group meetings and follow the format and style used in those.

On the other hand, if you are going to be the designated recorder for a series of meetings, then you should obtain guidelines from the organization involved. If such guidelines are not available, do some research and, in conjunction with the person appointed as chair, work out the style of minutes that you believe would best suit this particular group. You can look online for minutes templates to help you select what is best for your group. Some recorders take notes during a meeting and rewrite these into the proper format later; others find it more efficient to open their laptops and type onto the template as the meeting progresses. Make sure you check with the chair regarding the proper process for releasing the minutes. Some chairs will want to review your minutes before they are distributed.

Work with the chair for the meeting because an agenda (an outline, usually numbered in point form, of the things to be discussed) is enormously helpful to the person who takes minutes; the minutes will then follow the same headings as the agenda. The agenda usually is prepared by the chair, but for some groups, it may be your responsibility.

The following are the basic items for an agenda:

1. Call to Order

2. Approval of Agenda
   2.1 Addition 1 (list as many as required)
   2.2 ...

3. Approval of Minutes of Last Meeting(s); use sub-numerals if more than one

4. Business Arising from Minutes
   4.1 First item from minutes (list as many as required)
   4.2 ...

5. Officers and Committee Reports (e.g., chair, treasurer, committee heads)
   5.1 First report (list as many as expected to report)
   5.2 ...

6. Unfinished Business (e.g., items tabled or referred from previous meetings)
   6.1 First item (list as many as needed)
   6.2 ...

7. New Business (could have been identified to the chair before meeting or may be added to agenda at opening)
   7.1 First new item (list as many items as needed)
   7.2 ...

8. Approval of Date of Next Meeting

9. Adjournment

The minutes would generally follow the same format, but *Robert's Rules* identifies several points that must be covered for each set of minutes:

- name of the group (or committee or section of the group)
- kind of meeting (e.g., regular, special, board, committee)
- date and place of meeting and time meeting opened
- presence and name of the regular presiding officer (chair) and secretary or, in either's absence, of the substitute
- indication of who attended meeting (i.e., a statement a quorum was present, total number attending, or full list of names of those attending and those who did not attend)
- approval (with corrections, if any) of minutes of previous meeting—or, in some circumstances, their postponement until later (the latter may require a motion)

- all main motions, amendments, points of order, and appeals and whether these passed or failed or were withdrawn
- reports given by committee chairs (with names) or other individuals and any actions taken
- special announcements (e.g., related meetings, relevant actions by other groups)
- time of adjournment

Formats for minutes vary, depending on the group's wishes and the style designed by chair and recorder. Avoid using subjective descriptive adjectives (e.g., "J. O. Blow gave an *excellent* presentation ...."). Notes may be in point form or (more rarely) written in narrative paragraphs. Some groups call for minutes to be prepared in columns with titles showing the following: Item of business, Person designated as responsible, and Action required. Other groups have columns titled: Item, Points of discussion, and Action (including the name of the person responsible for taking action and reporting back). If you are taking minutes for a group, such as your students' association, you may want to set up your own template or standardized format in a laptop used at the meeting.

All minutes should be properly typed, signed, and preserved in an e-file, hard copy binder, or other suitable form for future reference by the group, its members, and appropriate others. Some groups are required by law to keep their minutes either permanently or for a specific number of years.

RESEARCH PAPERS, THESES, AND DISSERTATIONS

If you are in the final years of a baccalaureate program or in a program for your master's or doctoral degree, you may be asked to prepare a research paper; this is more advanced and sophisticated than the typical essay papers of your early years and represents another specialized route with many rules. We will discuss these briefly, but when you are in a master's or doctoral program, usually you will take a specific course on this kind of advanced writing.

The APA manuals provide an overview for research papers, which is also generally true for theses and dissertations. Another excellent resource is *How to Write and Publish a Scientific Paper* (eighth edition), by Barbara Gastel and Robert A. Day (2016); Day was the original author and the book is considered a classic reference.

As a route, a research paper (sometimes called a research report) follows many of the rules already described in this book for student papers and reports. Sometimes a thesis is actually a research report. To prepare these assignments, as with all other written communications, you need to implement the SMART essentials and follow the writing PROCESS.

A research paper describes the findings of your investigations and analyses; usually, the writer is the principal researcher or a member of the research team that planned and carried out the project. By the time you are asked to prepare a research paper, you will have read numerous research reports and articles, and you will have taken or will be taking a course on the development of a research project.

Most likely, the project itself will start with the development of a research question or problem. Students often agonize over the evolution of a good research question. An excellent place to find one is in a health care setting; ask staff from your discipline what problems they find in their day-to-day work and then pose one of those as a research question. For example, unit staff may ask if a daily drink of prune juice is effective in reducing the need for pharmaceutical laxatives and you could design a way of testing this with a large group of patients. Preparation of the research question itself is a major task; if you do a good job of it, you will find it much easier later to write the research article or report.

Do preliminary research on the question itself before committing to a project. Eventually, you will write an abstract summarizing the research question and get it approved before you begin the project. You may also need to write a funding proposal and perhaps even go through a research ethics review process. Once you start looking into background material for the project, you will write up a literature review. When you have done the review, you will need to identify the method that you are going to use in the written communication. Every step of the research process involves a new written communication. You may actually write up many of the stages as you proceed through the project. Once you have carried out the research, you are ready to prepare the final report.

Format of a Research Paper

Most research reports follow the traditional, rigid scientific method of organization, which has become known as IMRAD, an acronym for **I**ntroduction, **M**ethod, **R**esults, **A**nalysis, **D**iscussion. It follows the same format, with a few variations, as that already described for reports and student assignments. Many of the variations depend on the audience—the instructor for your course or the supervisor of your thesis committee. If you are in a graduate program, the department of graduate studies may have a specific set of guidelines for the format and presentation; obtain these before you begin work. However, in general, the following shows a basic format for a research paper, although the order of items will depend on the expectations of your audience:

- **title page**, which usually has rigid rules: it is longer and more formal in tone, and the title must accurately describe the contents of the paper so that it can be retrieved easily in a literature search; usually, there is no cover for a research paper, so the title page includes name(s) and title(s) of the author(s) or project team, as well as addresses, date, and other relevant material; you may need to supply keywords (see Chapter 3)
- **preliminary pages**, which include a table of contents; a list of tables, graphs, or illustrations; and perhaps a preface and acknowledgements
- **abstract**, which may be written last and summarize the project and findings, or may be written first and outline what the graduate candidate proposes to do (depending on your supervisor or faculty guidelines); abstracts for theses and dissertations differ slightly from those for student papers (see Appendix A) but are usually limited to 350 words for inclusion in an index of abstracts
- **body of the research paper**, which includes some or all these elements:
  - introduction (which may be labelled as such in a research paper; it includes history of or background to the project)
  - statement of the research question, hypothesis, or objectives of the study
  - literature review
  - research method(s) used (may include subsections on design, sample, data collection, and methods for analyzing data)
  - statement on human rights protection, research ethics review process, or other approvals needed
  - statement on limitations of the study (may be positioned after results or as a subsection under the conclusion)
  - results or findings (what you found out, including all statistical data or thematic analyses; statistical data may be summarized, with or without tables, and the full data set included as an appendix)
  - discussion or interpretation (your analysis of and comment on the findings; may require subsections in a long study)
  - conclusions (if the project reached any; they may be included under the discussion section)
  - recommendations or applications (if the project reached any; they may be included under the discussion section or under the conclusion section)
  - concluding section for the body of the research report (may be omitted if you let the conclusions and recommendations speak for themselves)
  - appendices (in a research paper or thesis, they come before the references and bibliography because usually you prepare any appendices)

- references and bibliography
- index (may be required)

Helpful Hints for Research Papers, Theses, and Dissertations

- If this is a student project, discuss everything with your instructor (or thesis committee) as early as possible in the project and regularly as you proceed.
- Preparation of these papers is usually a massive project, so break it down into small stages, with deadlines, and never leave it until the last minute.

ARTICLES

At some time in your career, you may want to write an article for a professional journal; health professionals often want to share good ideas with other health professionals. The basic SMART elements and the writing PROCESS will also help you to prepare a good article that has a chance of being accepted by the editor and published in a journal.

As you contemplate the SMART elements, carefully consider yourself as a source. Can you speak authoritatively? Would someone be interested in your views on the subject? You can write an article as a student as long as you provide a student's viewpoint or interpretation. If you have spent considerable time researching a specific topic and gathering data that are new and pertinent, then you can write about that with authority. If you are elected as an officer of an association, you may be able to write on behalf of the members of that association (if they agree). Just be sure you recognize your role in writing the article.

The route will be a certain journal, so you need to be familiar with that journal. Look at its guidelines and format to see whether your message will be appropriate. Once you look at professional journals as a possible author, you will discover there are many different kinds (e.g., research journals, general interest journals, specialty journals, newsletters, abstract journals) and that within any one journal there are often different kinds of articles (e.g., news items, letters to the editor, editorials, opinion articles, general articles, research articles, book reviews). Numerous professional health care journals are published, and journals in related fields (e.g., sociology, management, leadership) accept articles from health professionals. Which journal and which type of article would be best suited to your message? To see the range of professional journals, visit a large biomedical library or search a health-related journal database. You need to be aware that many "predatory journals" exist online and exploit health professionals. These entice potential authors to write for poor-quality and sometimes illegitimate journals; most charge publication fees to authors without providing editorial and publishing assistance or genuine peer review associated with legitimate publications.

You also need to consider the readership of the journal, which will eventually make up your audience. If your message is directed to physicians, it will not be accepted if you send it to a nursing journal; for example, *Canadian Nurse* is not likely to accept an article telling doctors that they need to write more legibly. Some journals are directed to all registered health care professionals in a particular region (e.g., journal published by a state association or union). Others have special audiences, such as hospital administrators (e.g., *Journal of Hospital Total Quality Management*) or those interested in pharmacy research (e.g., *Journal of Pharmaceutical Science*).

You can gain a good understanding of the readers by reviewing the information, usually in small print, on the masthead. The masthead will also give you other information, such as names of editors, address of the journal, its frequency of publication, its cost and whether it is sold by subscription or sent only to members, and, usually, whether it welcomes unsolicited manuscripts for review. Sometimes the masthead will tell you circulation numbers, impact factor, and whether it is open access. Some journals occasionally publish a page with information for authors and you can also search for submission guidelines on the journal's website; these advise you about length of articles that can be submitted, describe rules of the route, and mention the style guide to be followed. They also will suggest whether you should send a query letter to the editor before you submit your manuscript.

You will also learn a great deal about the route and the audience simply by reviewing several issues of the journal for which you want to write. When you first begin to write articles for professional journals, it is a good idea to submit to a journal that you read regularly. If you scan all issues for the past year, you will get a good idea of recent topics and whether the tone is formal (as in most research journals) or slightly less formal (as in journals for a general audience). You could note whether the journal tends to use short, catchy titles or longer, research-oriented titles. You could see whether each article opens with an abstract. You could determine the messages that get published. You could notice the length of most articles. You could check whether the journal uses photographs or not. All these points will affect how you eventually approach your message.

Most articles fall into one of these categories:

- research articles, which are similar to, but shorter than, research reports
- informational articles on procedures, processes, and techniques (often called "how to" articles)
- case studies, which describe in detail care of a patient (a typical or an unusual case)

- practice-based articles, which focus on interventions used to address specific patient care needs (sometimes called "from the field" write-ups, hands-on clinical care descriptions, or "practical practice")
- historical articles, which may or may not follow a special historical research format
- articles on current issues—called "opinion pieces"—that include in-depth analysis of views on a new or controversial matter
- editorials, which usually are solicited by journal staff from experts

We are not going to describe in detail the format and background for article preparation. Complete books and numerous articles on the internet deal with this topic. We are going to show you, however, a sample manuscript for a letter to the editor of a nursing journal written by a (fictional) student nurse with a brief covering letter (see Box 5.8). Both could be submitted by email.

This example illustrates many of the points relevant to longer articles.

BOX 5.8   Sample Manuscript Letter to the Editor (Cover Letter)

7135 Narrows Street
White Tusk, AK 12345

March 25, 2019

Judith Raines, Editor-in-Chief
The National Nurse
50 Broadway
New Rogers, NY 12345

Dear Ms. Raines

I hope *The National Nurse* will consider publishing the attached letter to the editor.

If you have any questions or concerns, you can reach me at my home number (902-555-0167); early evenings are the best times to reach me. You can also leave a message for me on email at a&r_onymous@bol.com .

Sincerely

Ann Onymous (Mrs. R. K.)
Third-year student
Balhousie University School of Nursing

Points to Note

Letters to the editor need to be formatted so that they can be handled like a manuscript. A published letter in a professional journal usually does not contain a street address, only the city; the covering letter gives your address, email address, telephone number, and other relevant details and is therefore attached to the typescript for the letter to be considered for publication.

BOX 5.8   Sample Manuscript Letter to the Editor—Cont'd

Networking Idea Letter to Editor — page 1

A Staff-and-Student Networking Idea

Opportunities for nursing students to network with practising registered nurses are vital but seem to be difficult to set up. However, RNs at Seal Cove District Hospital near White Tusk, Alaska, have involved students from the Balhousie Nursing Program in small, informal, practical network groups in a way that benefits both nurses and students.

For several years, staff nurses from the pediatric unit regularly met informally over coffee in the hospital cafeteria for one hour at the end of the day shift every other Thursday to exchange information on current nursing literature. Those who participated took turns reviewing current online journals and reporting to the group on articles of interest. Not all staff could attend every time, but several staff found the sessions valuable, and the meetings settled into a routine. The one-hour time limit was strictly observed.

About one year ago, these pediatric nurses invited students assigned to the ward to attend the meetings. The students proved enthusiastic participants, and some asked if they could continue to drop in after they finished on the unit. The staff nurses agreed, and the reading group has become larger, with three students interested in pursuing pediatric nursing becoming regular participants. These students sometimes know about proposed new pediatric research projects of interest to the staff group, who may wish to participate in the project. Students gain from the regular friendly contact with practising nurses and from hearing practical discussions related to the literature.

Furthermore, the students have reported the idea in other departments, and two other "journal clubs" have been set up at Seal Cove Hospital, one by nurses in the emergency department and one by the geriatric staff; several students from Balhousie take part regularly. Administration at the hospital has supported this informal continuing education project by supplying free coffee, tea, and juice for meetings of all three groups.

BOX 5.8 Sample Manuscript Letter to the Editor—Cont'd

The Boundary Health Unit in Seal Cove also has set up a "Literary Lunch Bunch" and invites students assigned to the unit to take part. Unfortunately, few students can continue this involvement once the community health assignment is over because the midday time conflicts with class schedules. At least one student, however, has been an off-and-on regular with this group for six months and now plans to follow a career in public health.

Nurses who participate in reading groups in other areas might want to consider including students. I know from experience that this form of networking is much appreciated.

Ann Onymous
Third-year student, Balhousie University
White Tusk, AK

Points to Note

Most articles and other items (e.g., letters to the editor, news items, book reviews, classified ads) are submitted electronically; this may be as a file attached to an email message or through an electronic management system. Check the guidelines to see what submission procedure to use. Generally, the typescript should be double-spaced, with typical wide margins and each page clearly labelled with a running head and the page number, just as you do with your student papers. Follow the style recommendations (e.g., about punctuation, capitalization, spelling) required by the journal. You do not need to have a title page; the cover letter takes on this role.

Note the short paragraphs, which make reading easier. Letters in journals or newspapers are usually set in narrow columns, where even a short paragraph will look long.

Letters are one of the most popular sections in any journal and get the attention of a lot of readers. If you can keep your message relatively short (as in the 412-word letter above), it likely would attract more readers than an article on the same subject.

The section for Letters to the Editor frequently has a word limit (often 450 words maximum); check the beginning and end of the section in the journal to see if length is mentioned. Even if the journal does not specify length, keep your letter as short as possible.

Helpful Hint About Articles

- The briefer the better: short articles stand a much better chance of being accepted for publication than do long ones.

POINTS TO REMEMBER

❑ Throughout your career you will need to prepare hundreds of written communications. Technology will continue to drive changes to style, format, presentation, storage, and distribution of these documents.

❑ During your career, you may also want and need to learn to communicate effectively with the public and other professionals through the media (including social media). This, too, involves special routes for special audiences. Ethical issues must be considered related to privacy, confidentiality, and protection of personal information and data. You need to think SMART there as well.

❑ So, although the formats described in these chapters will be useful to you, the most important things to learn from this book are application of the SMART elements of communication and use of the writing PROCESS.

❑ The SMART elements and writing PROCESS principles will last for your lifetime. Once you have learned how to use these principles, you will be on the road to growth as a writer, no matter how styles change.

REFERENCES

Asthma and Allergy Foundation of America. (2019). *What Are Latex Cross-Reactive Foods?* [website]. Retrieved from https://www.aafa.org/latex-allergy/

Emaze. (2018). *Create. Share. Emaze: Emaze your audience with gorgeous 3D and video effects that wow!* Retrieved from https://www.emaze.com/

Gastel, B., & Day, R. A. (2016). *How to write and publish a scientific paper* (8th ed.). Westport, CT: Greenwood Press.

Haiku Deck. (2019). *Beautiful presentations without the struggle.* Retrieved from https://www.haikudeck.com/

Kelly, K. J., & Sussman, G. (2017). Review and feature article: Latex allergy: Where are we now and how did we get there? *The Journal of Allergy and Clinical Immunology: In Practice, 5*(5), 1212–1216. https://doi.org/10.1016/j.jaip.2017.05.029

Keynote. (2019). *Beautiful presentations for everyone. By everyone.* Retrieved from https://www.apple.com/ca/keynote/

Library of Congress. (2018). *Congressional record.* Retrieved from https://www.congress.gov/congressional-record

Microsoft PowerPoint. (2019). Retrieved from https://products.office.com/en-ca/powerpoint

Mount Royal University. (2018). *Studying and writing effectively.* Retrieved from http://www.mtroyal.ca/AcademicSupport/ResourcesServices/StudentLearningServices/StudyingWritingEffectively/effective_presenting.htm

Office of Career Services Harvard University. (2019). *Resumes, CVs, cover letters.* Retrieved from https://ocs.fas.harvard.edu/resumes-cvs-cover-letters

Parliament of Canada. (n.d.). The debates of the House of Commons [Hansard]. Retrieved from https://openparliament.ca/debates/.

Prezi. (2019). Prezi. Retrieved from https://prezi.com/

Projeqt. (2018). *Dynamic presentations for a real-time world.* Retrieved from https://dmklee.com/projeqt

Robert, H. M., III, Robert, S. C., Evans, W. J., Honemann, D. H., & Balch, T. J. (2013). *Robert's rules of order: Newly revised* (11th ed.). Cambridge, MA: Da Capo Press/Perseus Books.

Simon Fraser University. (2017). *Avoiding plagiarism.* Retrieved from https://www.lib.sfu.ca/help/academic-integrity/plagiarism

Slidebean. (2018). *Slides, simple and beautiful.* Retrieved from https://slidebean.com/

Slidedog. (2018). *Freedom to present.* Retrieved from https://slidedog.com/

University of Hawaii: Maui College. (2018). *Stand and deliver: Planning a class presentation.* Retrieved from https://maui.hawaii.edu/tlc/home/learning-resources/stand-and-deliver-planning-a-class-presentation/

University of Kent. (2018). *Tips on making presentations.* Retrieved from https://www.kent.ac.uk/ces/sk/presentationskills.htm

University of Toronto Mississauga. (2018). *Resume and cover letter resources.* Retrieved from https://www.utm.utoronto.ca/careers/jobs/resume-cover-letter-resources

Visme. (2019). *Speak loudly. Speak visually.* Retrieved from. https://www.visme.co/

Zoho Show. (2019). *Slides, stories and ideas to inspire.* Retrieved from https://www.zoho.com/show/

6 LAST words on SMART communications

By now we hope you are convinced that you can be a good (or at least an effective) writer if you attend to the SMART elements and PROCESS steps. You know that as a health professional (both as a student and as a graduate) excellent writing skills are invaluable. Whether you need to write an essay to pass a course, craft a résumé to get a position, write an email to maintain a friendship, or draft minutes for a social club, you should be able to do so with confidence after reading the first five chapters of this book.

We have decided to leave you with some LAST words of encouragement and advice related to being a skilled writer as you embark on your studies and eventually on your professional career. Each letter in the acronym LAST introduces an associated word or phrase.

Love words and appreciate how to use them expertly in your writing. Carefully selected words, appropriate to the communication route, skillfully formatted, and meticulously edited, can help you get an A on your assignment or ensure you get a job interview because your résumé is perfect. Think about the words you select and the effects they have on others. Words are a writer's friend. You want to spend time with them, play with them, move them around to see how meanings change. Words are the building blocks of a writer's craft. Good writers spend time reading others' words and appreciating how they use words to convey meaning and message. A good way to learn to appreciate words is to read widely. You do not always have to read the classics to find interesting and exciting words; they can pop up anywhere. A poem by a young student named Steven on a blog by teacher Laura Hopping (2018) states, "Words have the most power / more power than any bomb ...."

Writing well can, and should, be fun! You may grit your teeth at this idea, but when writing skills become more natural to you, writing should become a pleasant activity. (Although you might not notice you are having fun when you are actually writing!) Writing gets a lot of negative vibes. Think of the negative stereotypes associated with writing: writer's block, penniless novelists living in drafty attics, and journalists who follow unethical routes to get stories. There are many advantages and positives outcomes to writing. An ancient Chinese saying goes: "The faintest ink is more powerful than the strongest memory." Yes, writing is fun (at least for us and, we hope, for you, too).

Consider a few reasons why writing can give you pleasure. First, you can create something from nothing. You begin with a blank page and craft something of meaning or use. You control what you create. You might do a poem or a story. You can generate a mood: you can choose a somber tone; you can select lighthearted words and write amusing anecdotes. You can even make up words (and then you, not APA, will decide how they are spelled). What a privilege it is to master words and skillfully mold them into something others might read and find enriching.

Writing is a great route for self-reflection. You can express your emotions, fears, and struggles through your written words; then you can share them or keep them just for your own review or even shred or burn them. This sort of writing can lead to healing and a healthier you, which may eventually lead to more joy in your life. Writing about your experiences leads to greater self-awareness and perhaps a new perspective on past events. It is much less expensive than therapy!

Love words and then choose your words, no matter the purpose, with great care.

Attitude is a seemingly intangible element of great writing, impossible to teach, yet clearly obvious, especially in written communications. Attitude is closely aligned with Tone in the SMART elements. You should be aware that your attitude may come through involuntarily in your writing. A positive attitude will catch the interest of your audience, while a negative attitude will limit readership (or put your instructor in a gloomy mood)! Your attitude (e.g., mood, voice, tone) may reveal latent feelings toward your subject to anyone who reads your paper, blog, or email. Are you angry, indifferent, excited, bored? Your writing reveals a lot about you, how you feel as you write, and your views about your topic. Check the attitude embedded in your work by watching where you drift off as you are rereading your work. Do you find any angry, lackluster, or dull elements that might turn a reader off? If so, take a second look at your word choices and see if you can adjust your attitude for a more positive outcome. Mind you, sometimes you have to write when you are not in a great writing mood, especially if your paper is due tomorrow.

Simple is powerful. Effective written communications are not long and rambling; instead they make a point in a pithy and concise way. Other S words—such as short, straightforward, and subtle—also apply to good informational writing. One way you can simplify your writing is to remove extraneous words (like *the*) to make your writing clearer. This important consideration usually arises during the Shine step in the writing PROCESS. Use punctuation skillfully to avoid excessive (and unnecessary) repetition. As we have explained several times already, however, clear, concise writing takes time. As letter writers frequently tell their friends: "I would have written you a shorter letter if I had time."

Tools are important to good writers. Just as a carpenter cannot build a house without a hammer and nails, a good writer cannot create an excellent product without writing tools. Finding just the right word to convey a subtle meaning or nuance is a challenge even for experienced writers. So indispensable tools include a good dictionary and a thesaurus. A scholarly dictionary—not just a cheap word book—usually gives several definitions and may give a history of the word (etymology), pronunciation, roots in other languages, grammatical information, and quotations illustrating correct use. A dictionary helps you discover overtones words can have, helps improve your vocabulary, and helps expand your world.

A thesaurus (online or hard copy) presents you with a selection of great words so that you can express exactly what you mean. Online versions give you quick access to options when you have trouble pinpointing the exact word you know you want. You do not just substitute another word to avoid repetition; selecting the perfect word clarifies and expands your idea. Never use a word unless you are positive of its meaning—and never use a word just to impress.

Other tools include online spell-checkers, grammar checkers, and your friendly computer. Google (or another search engine) can be a great writing aid if used skillfully. Technology provides you with other useful tools that may become indispensable depending on your genre of writing, your own writing weaknesses, or the type of route you use. For example, templates, such as those for business reports or minutes, can reduce writing time. Although technology is useful, you—a human—still need to make all the delicate editing decisions.

So, to sum up, we hope that this book will help you, and we wish you success with your written communications and a happy career as a health professional.

REFERENCE

Hopping, L. (2018). Hopping fun creations [Blog post]. Retrieved from
http://www.hoppingfun.com/blog.htm?post=996119

Today's students usually submit papers by electronic file, although some may still present their papers to the instructor by a traditional paper manuscript (hard copy). These general rules apply to both.

Most of your assignments will be prepared on a computer using a word-processing program. Ideally you should use a typeface that is clear and easy to read on a screen. If you submit handwritten papers (as in some journalling or conceptual mapping exercises), just take care that they are legible. Most standard settings on the word-processing programs on today's computers conform to the basic rules of the APA manuals. You may find it easier to follow the APA guidelines if you do **not** ask your computer to "auto-format" but set your headings and spacing yourself. Auto-format settings often use larger sizes of typeface or colours for headings, which are not appropriate for student papers. Take time to learn how to set margins, to use the tab and indent keys (especially the "hanging indent" commands), and to set headers and page numbers; such a learning investment will save you hours of reformatting as you work on your paper.

APA manuals have a section on student papers, theses, and dissertations; they say you (source) *may* deviate from the guidelines as the manuals are used to prepare journal articles (a specific route). APA manuals also stress that you should adhere to recommendations specified by your department or instructor (audience).

Our "rules" and the sample student paper in Box A.1 provide background and a more complete set of guidelines for introductory-level student papers in health disciplines. Please note that rules for theses and dissertations differ again; guidelines for some of the differences are provided in Chapter 5.

Select a standard, 12-point, serif font, such as Times New Roman (preferred), Courier, or Pica, for the text of the assignment (see Box 1.1 in Chapter 1). Use the same size typeface throughout the main parts of the paper, including headings and subheadings; do not change font sizes for those. The APA recommends using a standard font for the title page of articles, but note that requirements for preliminary pages, including the title page, may vary in your faculty. So you could, if your instructor allows, use a larger type for the title on the title page. When you begin to use figures and graphics in your assignments, you may use a sans serif font, such as Helvetica or Arial, because these save space and enhance visual presentation; you may even alter the font size (but keep it readable).

Some beginning students reduce or enlarge the font size or the line spacing in the body of the paper to help them meet page-length requirements asked for by an instructor in the assignment guidelines; take care, because instructors are familiar with this trick.

Use margins of at least one inch at the top, bottom, and left and right sides of the page. These standard margins are usually programmed into your word processor, although you can change them. Occasionally, your instructor will ask you to leave wider margins on hard copy assignments so that he or she can provide feedback. As always, an instructor's special requirements override all other style guidelines.

Double-space lines (even for handwritten papers) in the body of the paper; doing so makes it easy to read. Because your paper is a finished product in itself and not a manuscript being submitted to a publisher, you may choose to use single spacing for some parts of your paper. APA manuals advise you may use single spacing in tables, footnotes, and long quotations, and double-spacing in reference lists. However, your instructor may allow you to use single spacing in your references and bibliography (although then you must double-space between entries to make it easy to distinguish individual references). You may also choose to leave a space (double-double-space) before subheadings and in other places where it would improve the appearance of your paper (e.g., on the title page, after a title or a table, and before footnotes, or to avoid having a subheading on the bottom line of a page).

Number your pages in the top right-hand corner, using Arabic numbers, beginning with the title page. In the section on student papers, the APA manuals note that preliminary pages may be numbered with lower case Roman numerals except on the title page (as is done in the front of this book and in theses and dissertations); Arabic numbering then starts with a 1 on the first page of the body of the paper. Short student assignment papers probably will not have separately numbered sections, but papers should be numbered throughout starting with page 1 (even the title page). In the sample student paper that follows, the pages are numbered with Arabic numbers starting with the title page.

You should also use a "running head" (also called a "header"); this goes at the top left margin—on the same line as the page number, which is flush right. Headers (and footers) can be set using your word processing program and they go above (or below) page margins; once they are set, they are really helpful. The running head is brief (50 characters or less, including spaces) and usually consists of the first two or three words of the title of your paper. You should avoid using your name as the header (unless your instructor requests otherwise); some instructors prefer to mark papers without knowing the student's name, and later in your career, when you submit articles to journals, you do not use your name because articles are reviewed anonymously. You identify the words of your running head on the title page of your paper or first page by stating "Running head: WORDS FROM TITLE"; on all following pages just the running head is used (e.g., WORDS FROM TITLE). Note that you use capital letters for running heads.

Indent the first line of every paragraph one-half inch using the tab key. Certain passages in the text, such as long quotations (i.e., block quotations) and some lists, may also need to be indented; this is best done using the indent key or keys.

APA manuals do not provide guidelines for indenting annotations in an annotated bibliography (see Chapter 3), but the APA annotated reference list uses a standard half-inch indent followed by another two-space indent; in other words, the annotation is indented farther than the second line of the reference. This usually involves changing the spacing of the tab keys on your word-processing program. You may do this, or you may simply use two five-space indents, which is the common default setting for tabs on your program.

Most instructors prefer to mark papers on the computer as this allows them to give you a special kind of response right on your paper. They may use a yellow (or other) highlight to identify specific passages you need to work on, use "Track Changes" options (built into your word processing program) to redline (cross out) unnecessary words or phrases, or insert comment boxes to give you feedback.

You may want to check before the paper is due to be certain your word processing program is compatible with the one used by your instructor (i.e., that you can send a file and receive it back). Computers (e.g., tablets or mobile devices) may not send and receive files in a compatible format. If either you or your instructor cannot read the file, you may be able to send it from the campus learning centre or library as those computers are regularly updated and upgraded. You may also find that there are some problems if you use email to transmit a paper; email transmissions often alter the format, especially in relation to lines. Check the course syllabus and instructions and discuss electronic submissions fully with an instructor before assuming you can submit an electronic file at the last minute before the deadline. And always remember to keep a backup copy of your finished file.

The following pages show portions of a fictional student paper to illustrate one way that you might set up a short and relatively simple paper for your instructor. Remember, however, that you must think SMART. Some instructors (audience) might ask for different layouts. The information presented in some papers (message) might call for a more complex format (e.g., more subheads). If you are thoroughly familiar with APA style, you (source) might wish to amend this layout slightly to fit your views about a good presentation.

The following paper was written in response to this fictional request from an instructor in a Canadian nursing program:

Assignment 2 (due December 8, 2020)

Write a brief essay (about 1500 words or a maximum seven pages of text) in which you recommend reference materials that would be helpful to first-year nursing students. Use the most recent edition of the APA (2010) *Manual* as a guide for formatting your paper. Please supply an outline and a table of contents.

Write Tools 1

The Write Tools

by Glennis Zilm

Student Number: 98-76543

Assignment 2 (Date submitted: December 8, 2020)

Writing Skills Course E107x

University of Surrey

Instructor: Beth Perry, RN, BScN, PhD

email: gzilm@oohay.com

Write Tools 2

Table of Contents

Write Tools 3

The Write Tools: Outline

I. Introduction

short section introducing the paper and stating that students

need to have good writing tools (called "the write tools")

on hand to help them with their courses and giving my

recommendation for the best ones

II. Body of Paper

A. Dictionary (hard copy and online)

B. Grammar Resources

C. Style Manual (online preferably or hard copy)

– what a style manual is

– why it is needed

III. Conclusion

Write Tools 4

The Write Tools

Students who hope to do well in their courses need good

writing skills. Good writers usually have an array of "writing

tools" to help them. In particular, students need access to three

basic "write tools": dictionary resources, grammar resources, and

an approved style manual. In this paper, I give a brief overview of

these tools and why each is useful. I also recommend the ones I

believe students should own.

Dictionary Resources

A good, college-level dictionary is an essential tool for any

student writer—even if he or she uses a computer that has a spell-

checker built in. Dictionaries are much more than lists of words

spelled correctly.

Write Tools 5

They provide information on shades of meaning of
synonyms (e.g., character, personality, individuality). They
offer information on pronunciation of words (e.g., various
pronunciations of *lever*). They point out distinctions in
homographs, which are words that sound the same but have
different spellings and different meanings (e.g., *root, route*), and
homonyms, which are words that are spelled and sound the same
but have different meanings (e.g., *rose* [flower], *rose* [past tense
of *rise*]). They distinguish between various tones of meaning
(e.g., formal, informal, slang, derogatory, archaic). They provide
valuable information on how a word is used (e.g., as a noun or
verb or both). They may even provide information on the origins
of a word and the changes it has gone through during its history
(etymology). As Canadian poet A. M. Klein wrote in 1966: "To
know the origins of words is to know the cultural history of
mankind" (as cited in Colombo, 1974, p. 313).

Write Tools 6

Dictionaries often reflect the country of origin, such as those written and published in Britain or in the United States. Canadian students should own a Canadian dictionary; the *Gage Canadian Dictionary* (de Wolf, Gregg, Harris, & Scargill, 1997) is my personal choice. It was compiled by a group of distinguished Canadian lexicographers and has been revised and brought up to date to reflect current Canadian usage. The 1983 second edition (Avis, Drysdale, Gregg, Neufeldt, & Scargill, 1983) contains a wonderful essay on "Canadian English" originally written in 1967 by Professor Walter S. Avis, one of the original compilers and an expert on Canadian expression; this essay makes one proud of the depth and breadth of the Canadian language. As Avis (1983) wrote:

> The part of Canadian English which is neither British nor American is best illustrated by the vocabulary, for there are hundreds of words which are native to Canada or which have meaning particular to Canada. . . . Few of these words, which may be called Canadianisms, find their way

Write Tools 7

into British or American dictionaries, a fact which should

occasion no surprise. (p. xii)

Many courses require that a student writer use a specific

dictionary, such as *Merriam-Webster's Collegiate Dictionary*

(11th ed.) (2016), which is the dictionary and edition

recommended for use by the American Psychological Association

style manuals. However, publisher Merriam-Webster also

produces online versions of this dictionary, which can be updated

and revised easily so that the dictionary is current and often much

more useful than the hard copy version. Be sure that the word

processing program on your computer uses a complete version

that includes all the meanings and shades of meaning.

Grammar Resources

Even students who feel reasonably secure about their writing

skills will benefit by having a sound grammar reference resource

among their Write Tools. . . .

Write Tools 10

References and Bibliography

American Psychological Association. (2010). *Publication manual of the American Psychological Association* (6th ed.). Washington, DC: Author.

Avis, W. S. (1983). Canadian English. In W. S. Avis, P. D. Drysdale, R. J. Gregg, V. E. Neufeldt, & M. H. Scargill (Compilers), *Gage Canadian dictionary* (pp. xi–xiii). Toronto: Gage.

Avis, W. S., Drysdale, P. D., Gregg, R. J., Neufeldt, V. E., Scargill, M. H. (Compilers). (1983). *Gage Canadian dictionary*. Toronto: Gage.

Colombo, J. R. (1974). *Colombo's Canadian quotations*. Edmonton: Hurtig.

Day, R. A. (1993). *How to write and publish a scientific paper* (4th ed.). Phoenix, AZ: Oryx Press.

Write Tools 11

de Wolf, G. D., Gregg, R. J., Harris, B. P., Scargill, M. H.

    (Compilers). (1997). *Gage Canadian dictionary* (Rev. ed.).

    Toronto: Gage.

Merriam-Webster's collegiate dictionary (11th ed.) (2016).

    Springfield, MA: Merriam-Webster.

Northey, M., & McKibbon, J. (2015). *Making sense: A student's*

    guide to research and writing (8th ed.). Don Mills, ON:

    Oxford University Press.

Perry, B. (2020). *E107x Course Syllabus, University of Surrey*

    Department of English. Surrey, BC: University of Surrey

    Department of English.

HEADINGS

Headings are another matter of style that may differ in student papers. In recent APA manuals, the style for headings has been simplified: five levels of headings may be necessary in articles. APA recommends:

Level 1: **Centred, Boldface, Uppercase and Lowercase Headings** (no period)

Level 2: **Left-aligned, Boldface, Uppercase and Lowercase Heading** (no period)

Level 3: **Indented, boldface, lowercase heading.** (a paragraph heading, with initial cap, has a period, and the paragraph then runs on after the heading)

Level 4: ***Indented, boldface, italicized, lowercase heading.*** (similar to level 3 heading, but in italics)

Level 5: *Indented, italicized, lowercase heading.* (similar to level 4 heading, but not bold)

You can use only as many of these as you need, depending on the complexity of your content (shorter papers may only need two or three levels). Note these are guidelines and, if you are not required to use APA style, you may select the levels that suit the content of the article; for example, you may decide to use extra line spaces before a heading because you prefer that look.

You need to have the title of your paper centred at the top of the first page, but you do not use the subhead "Introduction" because it is assumed the beginning of the paper is the introduction. Notice that some text follows each subheading; only rarely are subheadings set together without some intervening text; two subheadings follow one another only within tables.

PARTS OF A PAPER (INCLUDING A SAMPLE STUDENT PAPER)

A formal student essay may contain some or all of these elements:

- cover page (or title page)
- table of contents or outline page
- abstract
- main text or body of paper
- references
- bibliography
- appendix or appendices

Many student papers, especially first-year papers, need only a cover or title page, the main text, and a reference list (or combined references and bibliography). Papers get more complex as you progress through your program, and theses and dissertations are the most complex of all (see Chapter 5 on these routes). How do you determine what is needed? First, check the course syllabus for instructions about the assignment; most instructors state their requirements there. If you are in doubt, ask. Remember to think SMART.

Cover Page

One of the most important items in the final draft of your paper is a good cover page or cover sheet. Sometimes called a title page, it goes at the front of your assignment. It is often a good idea to begin work on your title page—or at least on the title itself—as soon as you begin to plan your paper. The final draft of the cover page (during the shining-up stage) should include some of the following basic information: title of your paper, your name (unless your instructor specifies otherwise), your student number, name of the course (and section if the course is divided into sections), name of the university and department, instructor's name, and date the assignment was submitted.

You may wish to develop your own style for the cover page. Just be sure to include the essentials. And even if you are a wonder on the computer and can develop a colourful cover with large, beautiful fonts and borders, remember that this is a student paper in a professional discipline, not a document for sale. Fancy typefaces and graphics may give a different tone than you intended; some instructors do not like to receive a paper that looks as if you spent more time designing the cover than working on the content.

A catchy title is a great idea. It introduces your assignment and can provide, in a brief phrase or two, a capsule comment on your topic. The title should be clear and interesting. However, the title should relate to the content in your paper, so you may need a subtitle. For example:

Right Ways to Write:
Better Papers Mean Better Grades (subtitle)

A sample cover sheet—a plain, simple one—is shown in Box A.1. You may decide to format your cover differently, but this style is offered as a model.

Table of Contents Page or Outline

In short student papers, usually a table of contents page is not required. However, many instructors ask students to submit a table of contents or an outline—and that is because instructors know the importance of the O in the writing PROCESS; they want students to get into the habit of organizing and outlining. Furthermore, if your ideas do not flow smoothly from one section of the paper to another, a table of contents or outline helps the instructor to see your overall plan. In Box A.1, the Sample Student Paper, both a table of contents page and an outline page are shown.

Abstract

An abstract is a short, comprehensive summary of your paper. For journal articles, APA manuals recommend between 150 and 250 words. Some journals restrict the length to 75 to 100 words. An abstract is an essential component of most journal articles, and you will see many of them in your readings. An abstract tells readers what your article is about, what your conclusions are (briefly), and how these findings may be interpreted. Its main purpose is to assist researchers when they do literature searches and must review hundreds of articles. Abstracts often are included in online databases; potential readers can then usually tell whether they wish to obtain the whole article.

An abstract differs from an introduction, although the two are similar in content; even if you write an abstract, you still need an introduction. A main difference is that an abstract usually includes a statement about findings, whereas an introduction indicates the flow of the article to come and does not necessarily reveal findings. Students usually find it best to write the abstract after the body of the paper is in its final draft.

Some instructors, particularly those in senior years, ask students to write abstracts as a learning experience. APA manuals devote a section to describing what an abstract is; refer to that as a starting point if you are asked to write one. Whole books on abstracts are available, for example, the classic *Art of Abstracting* (Cremmins, 1996). You can also search the internet for newer, shorter articles and advice on abstracts, such as Tricia Leggett's (2018) article "Getting to the Heart of the Matter: How to Write an Abstract."

Another kind of abstract is that submitted to review committees by individuals (including students) who want to give an oral presentation (paper) or poster display at a conference; these abstracts are intended to tell the committee, and later the delegates to the conference, what the writer is prepared to talk about or display. These usually are written before the presentation or poster display is prepared.

Body of the Paper: Format

In Box A.1 we show the opening and closing pages of a short Sample Student Paper—a paper that probably would be about 1500 words long. You will note that there is a brief, one-paragraph introduction. The introduction indicates that the paper is divided into three sections, and then each section opens with a heading. Remember, too, that the introduction and the conclusion need to be the clearest and most memorable parts of your paper; see Chapter 2 for more information about this point.

If you look back at the table of contents and outline for this paper, you will see that only two levels of heading are needed: the title, which is repeated (per APA style) at the top centre of the opening page of the body of the paper; and one level of subheading.

The Sample Student Paper shows minor differences from the style recommended by the APA manuals for articles; however, it is consistent with advice given in the section that discusses student papers. In the section on student papers, the manuals make it clear that student papers— because they are "final" copies—may differ from manuscripts prepared for editors of APA journals. So, unless your instructor has provided specific guidelines telling you otherwise, you may wish to follow our Sample, which uses extra spaces before subheadings, among other minor style changes. In fact, you may even wish to single-space long quotations (which is not done in the Sample) and single-space tables. Tables are not shown in this Sample because students usually do not have to do them until later in their programs and because tables in student papers can differ widely. Tables in student papers usually can be done simply using the "Insert Table" option of your word-processing program.

The opening pages in the Sample illustrate two methods of formatting quotations within the body of the paper. The APA guidelines advise that if the quotation is less than 40 words, it should be included within the text paragraph. For longer quotations, the whole passage is indented (use format keys) one-half inch from the left margin (same spacing as the tab indent used for a paragraph). Note that an indented quotation is not enclosed in quotation marks. Look the sample paper over carefully; you may find many other small points that will be helpful to you as you format your own paper (e.g., where to position the period in relation to the citation in an indented quote).

References and Bibliography

The "References and Bibliography" page of the truncated Sample Student Paper in Box A.1 shows only a few of the references that might be included if the sample were a complete paper, but the ones included are enough to give you some ideas about the formatting of this section. Because this was to be a short paper (maximum 1500 words), the references and bibliography were combined, not presented separately; thus, there are books in the list that were not referred to in the paper.

Note that the References list always starts on a new page (because it is a separate section and not part of the main text or body) but that the subheading is in the same style as the subheadings in the main body of the paper. You might also wish to notice how the listing appeared in this section for the A. M. Klein quotation (taken from a secondary source).

CHECKLIST FOR STUDENT PAPERS (APA STYLE)

The following checklist reviews some points to keep in mind when shining up your paper:

- Use standard size pages 8½" × 11".
- Set at least one-inch margins at top, bottom, and left and right sides of all pages (these are usually the default margins).
- Justify the left margin but leave the right margin unjustified ("ragged" or "flush left").
- Use a standard 12-point typeface with serifs, such as Times New Roman, CG Times, Courier, or Pica.
- Double-space lines in the main text (and in most other parts of the paper unless other spacings would improve appearance and readability).
- Number all pages in the top right-hand corner, beginning with the title page.
- Identify your running head on the cover page and set it flush left on the same line as the page number, which is flush right; the running head then appears on every page.
- Read the paper aloud: Is it easy to read, or do you stumble anywhere?
- Check length of your sentences: Are there too many long sentences?
- Do too many sentences start the same way? Look especially for sentences with weak openings (e.g., "There are . . ." or "This is . . ." or "It was . . .").
- Check for improper use of first-person pronouns (*I, we, my, our, me, ours*).
- Check usage: Have you used jargon, slang, or clichés?
- Check sentence structure: Are too many sentences in the passive voice?

- Check style of your title, headings, and subheadings.
- Check spelling of any word about which you are not completely certain.
- Check use of capitals: Are they consistent? Do you have a reason for using the capital letters you used throughout your paper?
- Check punctuation: Have you used a comma before the word *and* in a series of three or more items? Do you have too many commas? Are there quotation marks where they are needed? Have you used apostrophes appropriately? Are there too many dashes and exclamation points (which signal an informal tone)?
- Proofread the finished, printed copy through a final time; do not change your content but make minor corrections.
- Keep a copy of your paper; even the best instructors occasionally misplace a paper.
- Always remember that your instructor's requirements outrank all other style guidelines.
- Think SMART.

REFERENCES

Cremmins, E. T. (1996). *The art of abstracting.* Arlington, VA: Information Resources Press.

Leggett, T. (2018). Getting to the heart of the matter: How to write an abstract. *Radiologic Technology, 89* (4), 416-418. Retrieved from http://www.radiologictechnology.org/content/89/4/416.extract

Note: Page numbers followed by *f* indicate figures, *t* indicate tables, and *b* indicate boxes.